Vitamins Can Kill Cancer

Reagan Houston, MS, PE

Infinity Publishing
West Conshoshocken, PA, USA
Phone: 877-289-2665
www.bbotw.com

Cover Design by Michael Gaffney, Young Creative Associates, Inc., Hendersonville, North Carolina

ISBN 0-7414-3253-6

Published by:

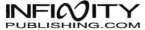
PUBLISHING.COM

1094 New DeHaven Street, Suite 100
West Conshohocken, PA 19428-2713
Info@buybooksontheweb.com
www.buybooksontheweb.com
Toll-free (877) BUY BOOK
Local Phone (610) 941-9999
Fax (610) 941-9959

Printed in the United States of America

Printed on Recycled Paper

Published May 2006

This book is dedicated with thanks to:

Abram Hoffer, M.D., Ph.D., F.R.C.P. (C)
for his pioneer work, advice and suggestions;

Townsend Letters for Doctors and Patients
for publishing much of my work with some of it
republished here;

My wife, Mary, for support and proofreading;

Pardee Hospital, Hendersonville, NC
for allowing me to facilitate the Prostate Cancer
Support Group and select speakers;

Librarian Chris Kersten
for innumerable magazine reprints; and

God
for help, guidance and motivation.

DISCLAIMER

The following is a compilation of scientific studies and papers describing research and opinions on the health benefits of vitamins and nutritional supplements in the prevention and treatment of various human cancers. This book is educational and is not intended as medical advice, as the author is not a physician. This book contains certain of the author's opinions and is not intended as a substitute for recognized cancer treatment modalities or the advice of your physician. The author's objective is to provide readers with a summary of certain scientific literature so that they can ask their doctors about and draw their own conclusions concerning the role of vitamins in the treatment and prevention of cancer. Every individual's physical condition and response to vitamins is unique. The opinions contained in this book have not been evaluated by the U.S. Food and Drug Administration.

Preface

by Dr. Abram Hoffer, MD, PhD, FRCP(C)

About 1790, 40 years after Sir James Lind, MD, proved that giving scorbutic sailors oranges and lemons cured them, the British Admiralty ordered that lemon juice be given all sailors in the Navy. However, during that intervening 40 years, hundreds of thousands of sailors died a horrible death from scurvy. Why did it take so long to act? Luckily for the British they did not wait another 40 years.

The lemon juice saved England from being invaded by Napoleon. For, at that time, the French fleet was too sick to stand out to sea long enough to be an effective navy. They probably had heard about lemons too, but did not act upon this information.

This 40-year delay is almost a must for all new paradigms in medicine. It takes two generations of physicians to give up the old and accept these new paradigms. In modern times it may take even longer, because the medical profession is much more organized and under the thumb of their leaders. Also, nutrition has always had a rough time being accepted onto medicine. It was beginning to come of age just before the War, during the golden age of vitamin discovery. During this age Nobel Prizes were given.

Goldberger, who discovered the cause and cure of pellagra, did not get one: the medical profession was convinced that pellagra was an infectious disease caused by the bite of a horse fly.

It is taking an equally long time for the cancer establishment to accept that nutrition and nutrients play an important role in the cause of cancer, and in its prevention and treatment. It accepts that vitamins like vitamin C and vitamin E, both natural antioxidants, are valuable—but only if they are present in food in small amounts and not if they are supplements. The cancer establishment has promulgated an amazing number of factoids about vitamins, including the one rigidly held by almost all oncologists that vitamin C will decrease the therapeutic effect of chemotherapy and radiation, in spite of an overwhelming amount of clinical and research data showing that this is not true.

In 1971 Dr. E. Cameron was examining the anticancer properties of vitamin C at his hospital in Scotland, the Vale of Leven. Later he was joined by Dr. Linus Pauling. The evidence was plausible, but double blinds had overtaken the scientific part of the medical profession, and only double blinds would thereafter be considered of any value. I found this interesting as the first psychiatric double blinds were done under my direction in Saskatchewan, starting in 1952, when we studied the effect of vitamin B-3 in treating schizophrenia successfully. But I was also among the first to point out that it had major defects. It should never have become the gold standard of medical research, and I hope it will soon die a natural death.

If we must wait an additional 50 years before Cameron's findings will be accepted, will we have to wait until 2021? Should we really have to wait this long? In contrast to chemotherapy which is inherently and by design very toxic, vitamin C, even in very large doses, is not toxic. It kills only cancer cells.

I published my clinical data to record what had happened to my patients hoping this would stimulate more interest, and I believe it has.

I hope that a personal and well-reasoned account such as this one will shorten the time required. Maybe I am too optimistic.

January 4, 2006   A. Hoffer MD (Ret.) PhD FRCP(C)

Introduction

In 1969 The National Cancer Institute found that vitamin C killed cancer cells without harming normal cells. In 2005 the National Institute of Health repeated the successful NCI tests. Abram Hoffer,[1] M.D., PhD., and other doctors have developed vitamin C into a clinically tested cancer therapy using standard supplements of vitamins A, B, C, D and E plus selenium and zinc. *He helped hundreds of patients with many types of cancer live longer and with less pain.*

The mainline therapies for cancer—surgery, radiation, chemotherapy and hormones—work quite well and we should continue them. However, they weaken the body. Many clinical tests show that strengthening the body can greatly improve the results of using these mainline therapies. Vitamins and similar supplements have helped many cancer patients with various types of advanced cancer live many times longer than patients not strengthening their bodies.

Vitamins are tested, safe and effective. Because of their obvious safety and effectiveness, many believe that randomized and double blind tests are probably not needed for vitamins.

Irwin Stone[2] said that "the cancer problem has been solved, and all that is needed now is routine large-scale tests to verify this conclusion." These tests have been run and are reported here.

The author is a chemical engineer. He was diagnosed with an early but agressive type of prostate cancer. After an initial PSA of 8.1 and a Gleason of 6, he used vitamins and triple hormone therapy for about a year and then Proscar plus vitamins for the next 8 years. His cancer is nicely in remission with a PSA of 0.3. A normal PSA is 4.0 or less. He has never had chemotherapy, surgery or radiation of any kind. This is written in love to help others who may have cancer. He has no financial interest in any product or supplement mentioned here except book sales.

Reagan Houston, 600 Carolina Village Road, #165
Hendersonville, NC 28792
www.cancertherapies.org
h@cancertherapies.org

Vitamins Can Kill Cancer

Table of Contents

Section One

Vitamins, Cancer and Hope

Surgery, chemotherapy and radiation are good, standard cancer therapies but even with these, one-third of cancer patients die in five years.[3] Can we make these therapies more effective? Abram Hoffer, M.D., Ph.D[1]. a physician who had earned his Ph.D. studying vitamins and is the author of *Vitamin C and Cancer,* chose diet and vitamins to help patients live longer and to combat the body weakening caused by regular therapies. Hoffer, a psychiatrist, received his first cancer patients because they were depressed. One of these early patients had pancreatic cancer. Because the tumor at the head of her pancreas was inoperable, a bypass was installed. Her doctor offered no hope. He said she would be dead in three months.

But she had hope. She knew that Norman Cousins, *Anatomy of an Illness,* had recovered after his doctors had given up. Cousins had used 15,000 mg/day of vitamin C. Hoffer gave her vitamin C at 35,000 mg/day plus other supplements. Seven months later a CT scan showed no sign of cancer. Five years later, she decreased her daily dose of vitamin C. Twenty years after her terrible prognosis, she died at age 79. Even pancreatic cancer has been controlled! Yet, the American Cancer Society[3] reports that 96% of pancreatic cancer patients die within five years.

Hoffer's Multivitamins

Beginning in 1978, Hoffer[4,5] started a 15-year test on 134 advanced cancer patients. His approach was to counter the weakening effects of the cancer, surgery, radiation and chemotherapy by strengthening the body and the immune system. His early vitamin regimen[5] has been modified to give Table 1.1.[6] He recommends a diet low in meat, very low in sugar but high in fruits, vegetables and water.

Table 1.1. Dr. Hoffer's Average Regimen[6]
Use surgery, radiation and chemotherapy in moderation.

Beta carotene,	30,000 IU
Vitamin B complex	B-50 to B-100
Vitamin C	12,000 mg
range	3,000 – 40,000
Vitamin E,	300 IU
Selenium	600 mcg
Zinc	60 mg

Some patients received more B-3, vitamin A at 10,000 to 50,000 IU, and beta carotene up to 75,000 IU. Calcium and magnesium were occasionally included. Pills are taken each day in 3 divided doses with meals. The vitamin C may be taken as pills, powder or as sodium ascorbate.

Hoffer[7] has improved his average regimen by adding vitamin D3 at 4,000 to 6,000 IU, Coenzyme Q10 at 300 mg and a combination of curcumin 3,000 mg with bioperin 15 mg. As a major change, he recommends that patients receive 100,000 mg of sodium ascorbate by IV daily. He says "In many cases this kind of very safe chemotherapy...I think would bring most cancers under control pretty quickly."

Hoffer, born in 1917, retired after 2005.

To all of his cancer patients, Hoffer offered the vitamin regimen, diet and hope based on the results with earlier patients. Those who accepted vitamins thus had the advantage of vitamins, diet and hope compared to those who rejected vitamins. Self-selection is typical of real life but not ideal for statistical evaluation.

What Types Of Cancer?

Hoffer has treated over thirty types of cancers with impressive results, Table 1.2. Most of his patients had advanced cancers that could not be helped by surgery, radiation or chemotherapy. For example in his test group, those who refused vitamins lived a median of 2.6 months. Those who accepted vitamins lived 45 months or 17 times longer. All 32 of the breast cancer patients had surgery, radiation and/or chemotherapy. The median life of these very sick patients who chose to take vitamins was 70 months while those without vitamins had a median life of only 3.7 months.

Table 1.2. Median Survival of Hoffer's Patients with Various Types of Adv. Cancer, Months[4,5]

Type of Cancer	With Vitamins	Without Vitamins
Breast	70	3.7
Uterus	99	4.0
Ovary	16	3.6
Lung	17	2.0
Pancreas	40	2.4
All 30 types	45	2.6

Hoffer's vitamin therapy "has given [his patients] more energy, has improved depression and anxiety, has created a sense of well being, *has eased pain and has often eliminated pain entirely.*"[1]

As reported by Hoffer, Pauling said, "The cancer death rate could be reduced by 25% of its present value...if a reasonable multivitamin regimen were to be followed regularly by every person."

Cameron's Vitamin C Regimen

Dr. Ewan Cameron, MB, ChB,[8] Senior Consultant Surgeon in Scotland, described his first very advanced cancer patients in 1971. "They responded dramatically indeed, being converted from a hopeless, terminal 'dying' situation into a hopeful 'recovering' situation." After 8 years and treating 500 terminal patients of many types of cancer, Cameron concluded that vitamin C is not a miraculous cure but a major step forward.

Instead of a handful of common vitamins such as Hoffer used, he started his patients on vitamin C only. He administered vitamin C in the form of sodium ascorbate and mostly at 10,000 mg/day intravenously for two weeks along with oral vitamin C continuously. Cameron used vitamin C by IV for 33 of his first 50 patients. Thus, 17 patients received only oral vitamin C in large doses.

His vitamin-taking patients lived four times longer than similar patients at the same hospital who were not given vitamins. Cameron joined with Dr. Linus Pauling, a double Nobel Laureate, to publish the results in *Cancer and Vitamin C* in 1993.

Vitamin C comes in several forms. Ascorbic acid is the common pill. Sodium ascorbate is nearly tasteless in solution and calcium ascorbate is preferred by some doctors. Cameron and a few other doctors report "ascorbic acid" when they mean sodium ascorbate. Ascorbic acid is too acid for intravenous injection.

Many other doctors have also used vitamin C as cancer therapy and published their results. Irwin Stone, D.Sc.[9] author of *The Healing Factor: Vitamin C against Disease*; Robert Cathcart, M.D.[10] a physician in Los Altos, California; Fukumi Morishige, M.D.[11] in Fukuoka, Japan and Hugh Riordan, M.D.[12] in Wichita, Kansas, successfully used vitamin C in the form of intravenous sodium ascorbate. Hoffer was able to successfully use oral vitamin C by including vitamin E and other vitamins.

Other Regimens

Drs. Edward Creagan,[13] and Charles Moertel[14] used ascorbic acid at 10,000 mg/day without success. Creagan's randomized test used patients whose immune system had been decimated by prior chemotherapy. Moertel administered vitamin C for an average of only 2.5 months although the test lasted over 14 months. Also, they did not administer IV sodium ascorbate nor follow Cameron's or Hoffer's regimens. Dr. Mary L. Lesperance[15] selected a portion of Hoffer's breast cancer patients for evaluation. She chose patients who avoided vitamin E and E succinate and control patients who were less sick than the test patients. Her test patients did not live longer than the controls. The regimens developed by Creagan and Moertel showed that some regimens do not work. They do not show that all regimens for vitamin C do not work.

Vitamin C Is Safe

Many people have taken 30,000 mg/day for years. Several doctors[10] have given 200,000 mg/day by IV. Some claim that vitamin C "might" cause kidney stones although doctors who give large doses of vitamin C rarely if ever see stones in these patients. Ascorbic acid can make the urine acidic to dissolve some stones.

Excessive vitamin C can cause diarrhea. People with cancer can frequently take and tolerate 30,000 mg/day while well people have a typical limit of 3,000 to 10,000 mg/day. If people on therapeutic doses of vitamin C develop diarrhea, the dose should be reduced. Actually, diarrhea is a useful blessing because it provides a simple measure of the proper dosage for each individual. Hoffer's patients who took from 3,000 to 40,000 mg/day illustrate the wide range of dosages for individual cancer control. Humans cannot make the vitamin C they need although most animals can. A 160-pound goat can make 13,000 mg/day—a reasonable dose for people with cancer. Hoffer advised his patients to continue the high vitamin doses indefinitely. Table 1.3 includes some of the precautions, side effects and alternatives listed by Riordan.[12] However,

Cameron and Hoffer did not report that they followed the precautions in step 5.

Table 1.3. Precautions with High-Dose Vitamin C

1. Build up the dose slowly by about 1,000 or 2,000 mg/day to minimize diarrhea and other problems.
2. If necessary, decrease the dose slowly to allow the body to adjust.
3. Vitamin C—especially ascorbic acid—may cause gas, upset stomach or skin itch. If this problem occurs, consider using sodium ascorbate or calcium ascorbate.
4. Excess sodium intake from sodium ascorbate is possible. Consider using calcium ascorbate or ascorbic acid.
5. Some people have a rare immune deficiency of glucose-6-phosphate dehydrogenase enzyme. These people may not be able to take large doses of vitamin C without getting acute anemia.
6. For their own safety people should work with a doctor knowledgeable about vitamins. All people may not be able to use high doses of vitamin C.

J.K.'s Vitamin C Regimen

As quoted in a letter to Dr. Albert Szent-Gyorgi, Dr. Irwin Stone[16] had a friend, J.K. who took massive amounts of vitamin C to control his metastasized prostate cancer.

"J.K. was diagnosed in May 1973 and received the usual high-risk surgery and radiation. In November 1977 a bone scan indicated the cancer had spread to the pelvic bone. At that time he was declared terminal with about one year to live. In January 1978 he started taking laetrile and 2 grams of ascorbic acid. After 10 months the cancer was still growing, so he modified his therapy to ascorbate orally at 24 grams per day. The cancer continued to grow and a new pelvic tumor was found as well as a tumor in his lung. In May 1979 he increased his ascorbate intake to 80 grams per day and at this level there was no cancer growth for the next 6 months. During the next 2 1/2 years the cancer was under control and it grew only when he reduced his ascorbate intake to less than 80 grams a day or he went off his diet (no beef, no candy, etc.) but stayed at 80 grams per day."

At this ascorbate intake, some tumors regressed or grew only very slowly. In 1982 J.K. was under great stress both at work as a chemist and patent attorney and at home. He increased "his ascorbate intake to 130 to 150 grams per day! He has been taking an oral dose every hour of 5 to 10 grams of a mixture of nine parts sodium ascorbate plus one part ascorbic acid dissolved in water. These doses were well tolerated and within bowel tolerance and he has had no trouble from diarrhea except just a little when he reduced the 150 grams a day to 130 grams."

Stone reported that J.K. felt great most of the time, worked every day and was living a fairly normal life. Orthodox medicine predicted his death by November 1978 but he apparently died seven years later on December 2, 1985.

At one time J.K. had an ascorbate blood level measured at 35 mg/deciliter. Normal blood levels are about 0.4 to 1.2 mg/dl. Riordan[12] found that 5 to 40 mg/dl were required to kill most or all types of cancer cells. Thus J.K.'s oral vitamin C regimen may equal the IV regimen of Riordan. Obviously, the high blood level reported for J.K. should be checked. One mg/dl equals 57 micromols.

How Vitamins Work

When vitamin C of any type acts as an antioxidant and neutralizes free radicals, it produces dehydroascorbate, DHA, an oxidant. Normal cells need and take in DHA. The DHA is then converted to ascorbate and hydrogen peroxide, H_2O_2, by an oxidation/reduction process. Normal cells safely neutralize excess H_2O_2 by a reaction with catalase.

DHA may be the key to vitamin therapy. Dr. L. Benade[17] et al at the National Cancer Institute found that, in cultures, vitamin C selectively destroyed cancer cells by generating excess intracellular H_2O_2. Cancer cells are less able than normal cells to neutralize H_2O_2 because they are deficient in catalase. Dr. David B. Agus[18] et al reported that cancer cells have extra glucose channels that rapidly bring in glucose and excess DHA. Cancer cells are defective in that they cannot fully distinguish between glucose and DHA. This may explain why vitamin C is safe in large doses for normal cells but toxic to cancer cells. The good results of Cameron and Hoffer with humans confirm the 1969 lab tests at the National Cancer Institute.

Benade's test was repeated at the National Institute of Health in 2005 by Dr. Q. Chen[19] and co workers in Dr. Mark Levine's group. Ten types of cancer cells were killed in cultures by vitamin C (sodium ascorbate) at concentrations attainable with IV in humans. Four types of normal cells were unaffected by much higher concentrations of vitamin C. Based on a different test method than Benade, Chen attributed cancer cell death to H_2O_2 generated outside the cell membranes rather than inside. H_2O_2 can permeate cell membranes. Thus both research groups concluded that H_2O_2 selectively killed cancer cells.

Chen noted that ascorbate "ironically initiates pro-oxidant chemistry and H_2O_2 formation." Levine's group has started a phase I safety trial on vitamin C. The work of Hoffer[1] is relevant to any future phase III trial.

High-dose vitamin C appears to act as an antioxidant in most of the body but as a cancer-killing oxidant within cancer cells.

John Boik[20] discusses the formation of H_2O_2 by vitamin C. He expects vitamin C to be helpful but not therapeutic at high dosages. He presents another view of how vitamins might kill cancer. He lists seven traits that distinguish

---

Table 1.4.

Seven Traits of Cancer and Therapeutic Vitamins

1. Defective DNA or bad genes
   Vitamins A, C, D, E and selenium

2. Abnormal growth factors within the cells
   Vitamins A, C, D, E calcium and selenium

3. Abnormal growth factors outside the cells
   Vitamins A, B6, B12, C, D, E and selenium

4. Excess growth despite surrounding cells and tissue
   Vitamins A, C, D, E and selenium

5. Abnormal blood-vessel growth, angiogenesis
   Vitamins A, C, D, E and selenium

6. Spread of cancer to new locations
   Vitamins A, B12, C, D, E and selenium

7. Ability to hide from the immune system
   Vitamins A, E, zinc and selenium.

---

cancer, Table 1.4. He describes how various vitamins combat each of these traits.

Hoffer's vitamins fight each of the traits with at least four vitamins and minerals. Vitamin C combats 6 of the 7 traits listed by Boik. Cancer mutates as it tries to survive but vitamins can continue to combat each trait.

Based on the long-term experiences of Hoffer and Cameron, and the need for most types of advanced cancer to feed on glucose, cancer mutation may not be a problem with vitamin C.

Hoffer's regimen included multiple vitamins. He recommended[21] vitamin C as ascorbic acid pills, as ascorbic acid powder or as sodium ascorbate powder. The latter two were often combined into water or fruit juice to make a tasty drink. Cameron's patients took oral vitamin C as sodium ascorbate solution, Table 1.5. Intravenous sodium ascorbate can be made as Cathcart[22] indicated.

Hoffer prefers that most or all of the vitamin E be in the form of d-alpha tocopherol succinate. This is commonly called vitamin E succinate or dry vitamin E and is available in health food stores. The vitamin E succinate may be significant since it limits cancer growth by regulating several genes. Vitamin E and E succinate have shown only minor cancer-killing power by themselves but may be of great help with vitamin C.

Table 1.5. Sodium Ascorbate Solution

Ascorbic acid .... 167 gm
Sodium bicarbonate .... 80 gm
 (baking soda)
Water and juice to .... 1,000 ml

Fifteen ml taken four times a day preferably with meals provides 10,000 mg/day of ascorbate. The refrigerated solution has a shelf life of about one month. The water solution has almost no taste. Add water first and then juice to minimize foaming.

Hickey and Roberts[23] in their excellent book *Ascorbate, The Science of Vitamin C,* 2004, carefully explain the basic science and delve deeply into the controversy of vitamin requirements and therapy results. They list several references that attempt to explain the mechanism by which vitamin C controls cancer. The important point is that vitamin C does combat cancer with excellent success.

Vitamin Acceptance

In 1973 Cameron reported on a successful clinical test of vitamin C for 50 and then 100 cancer patients. However, the medical community requires that new cancer therapies pass large, randomized and preferably double blind tests. Is this reasonable? Surgery, radiation and chemotherapy were each accepted in desperation without randomized tests against each other. Neither radiation nor chemotherapy can be given randomized, double blind tests versus each other because of the obvious and debilitating side effects. These therapies were accepted based on historic experience. To require vitamins to pass tests that radiation and chemotherapies have not and cannot pass demonstrates questionable logic. Perhaps it is reasonable to disregard the so called requirement for randomized and double blind tests for vitamins. Surgery, radiation and chemotherapy were accepted without randomized and double blind tests.

Hickey gives a thorough review of how to evaluate a proposed therapy. A few simple questions are sufficient:
1. Has it helped others?
2. Is it safe?
3. Can I continue known therapies?
4. Might it help me?

With regard to vitamins, the answer is yes on all questions. The new question becomes, *"Doctor, why are you **NOT** giving me high-dose vitamin C"?*

There are reasons that oncologists don't administer high-dose vitamin C, but are they good reasons? Many doctors say vitamin therapy is untested. Hoffer has treated over

1,300 patients in 25 years. Cameron has treated over 500 patients and Morishige 99, plus untold others by Stone, Cathcart and Riordan. Creagan and Moertel objected to vitamin C but did not report any harm from it. Many believe radiation was accepted with far fewer tests than vitamins, and for a shorter period.

Many doctors object to people taking antioxidants simultaneously with radiation or chemotherapy because they believe that the vitamin C, acting as an antioxidant, "might" protect the cancer cells. However Davis W. Lamson,[24] M.S., N.D., summarized thirty-six clinical tests where antioxidants were used with radiation or chemotherapy. The antioxidants were helpful in thirty-one cases, neutral or possibly helpful in five and adverse in none. He found that antioxidants are generally helpful with radiation and chemotherapy.

Judith O. Stoute[25] reviewed 44 articles regarding the use of vitamin C with chemotherapy. She found 36 positive studies or reviews, one neutral study, 2 negative reviews and 4 responses to the negative reviews. She concluded that vitamin C can generally be used with chemotherapy. Because vitamin C, radiation and some chemotherapies appear to kill cancer by a similar mechanism, vitamin C can generally be used with radiation and chemotherapy.

As explained earlier, vitamin C can be an antioxidant in most of the body but a cancer-killing oxidant in cancer cells.

Oncologists are trained in the use of mainline therapies. Because of peer pressure and mandates of state medical boards, they are frequently not allowed to recommend "unapproved" therapies such as vitamin C. They are likewise hesitant to recommend doctors or patients who know about vitamins as therapy. Most doctors knowledge-able about vitamins are not allowed to treat cancer, but they can recommend vitamins to strengthen people who have cancer. This narrow distinction is important and most useful.

A patient who wants to use vitamins can ask his family doctor (or a nutrition-knowledgeable doctor) for vitamins to strengthen his body. He should be careful about asking for vitamins to control cancer, as the doctor may have to refuse this request. These doctors should also know about exercise and diet. A poor diet can make cancer grow even with a good vitamin regimen. Doctors who can assist cancer patients with nutrition and vitamins may be located at The American College for Advancement of Medicine (www.acam.org) or in Dr. P. Quillin's book.[26]

Patients need oncologists and their extensive know-ledge. However those who want to use vitamins to augment regular therapies probably must work with a second doctor knowledgeable about vitamins as a team member with the oncologist. A patient who wants to use vitamins can ask his family doctor for vitamins to strengthen himself. He should not ask for vitamins to control the cancer. However, all physicians involved with the cancer patient's care should be fully informed about all treatment choices made by the patient, including the use of vitamins.

Randomized tests

Most doctors require randomized tests for chemotherapy drugs. Why? The Cancer Chemotherapy National Service Center was established in 1955 by the National Cancer Institute. They decided that test compounds should generally be lethal at doses greater than 500 mg/kg of body weight. This decision assumed that all chemotherapies would be toxic, a decision made with no sound basis. The decision effectively eliminated vitamin C from testing. Later in 1969 when Benade, at the National Cancer Institute, reported that vitamin C safely killed cancer cells but not normal cells, the decision became even more questionable. The decision meant that extensive laboratory, animal and human tests would be required. A dose suitable for some patients could be fatal for other patients. Because of the required toxicity most chemotherapies have a narrow margin between cancer death and patient death. These tests cost many millions of dollars since many compounds fail late in the testing process. The tests of hundreds of patients had to be carefully analyzed by statistics. The high cost of these tests means that the drug companies would test only patentable compounds.

Vitamin C, a natural compound, is not patentable. As noted earlier, randomized tests on vitamin C by Creagan and by Moertel did not show Vitamin C to be helpful. This is understandable since neither of their tests was run following the procedure recommended by Cameron and Pauling. Their claim that vitamin C was useless toward cancer applies only to their regimen. The government has refused to properly test vitamin C.

Drug companies, in fairness to their stockholders, cannot run expensive tests on non-patentable vitamins. However an interested individual or institution could repeat Hoffer's test regimen, especially with historical rather than randomized controls.

Because vitamin C does not fit the toxicity requirements of the government, many believe that vitamin C need not require randomized testing. As a crude comparison, vitamin C is much like castor oil:

It is safe.

It works.

It is self-limiting on dosage.

Based on the successes of Cameron and Hoffer, the Service Center's decision may have been a billion dollar mistake.

Cameron's clinical trial (even with retrospectively matched controls) is convincing because the vitamin-taking patients lived four times longer than those not receiving vitamin C. Hoffer's multivitamin detailed results are also convincing. The appendix shows individual results for each type of cancer for 134 patients in the study. Many doctors have used high-dose vitamins for cancer therapy— 1,300 patients by Hoffer and 500 by Cameron. They believe that vitamins for cancer therapy are sufficiently tested that they can now be used with proper medical supervision.

As Hickey points out, the benefits of ascorbate therapy clearly outweigh the risks.

Patient Options

Patients in a terminal or palliative hospice situation might well consider ascorbate vitamins. For them, the oncologist realizes that surgery, radiation and chemo-therapy have helped as much as they can and doctors knowledgeable about vitamins are available. Terminal patients are frequently willing to try experimental therapies.

These terminal patients often enter experimental clinical trials. In these tests half of the patients often get a placebo and thus are not helped. Vitamins are safer and offer more hope to terminal patients—hope based on clinical trials of over a thousand people.

Patients with an initial cancer diagnosis might also consider Cameron's or Hoffer's vitamin therapy under proper medical supervision. This situation is less tested, but general experience says that treatments started early often work better than the same treatment given later.

Vitamins without Radiation and Chemotherapy

Can vitamins lengthen the lives of patients who do not receive radiation or chemotherapy? Surgery for operable cancer is usually advisable to remove all or almost all of the cancer. The body then has less cancer to fight. Radiation aims to kill cancer locally while chemotherapy works throughout the body. Both therapies are poisons that also kill healthy cells. An unfortunate disadvantage for most oncologists is that they have only surgery, radiation, chemotherapy and occasionally hormones as tools to fight cancer. When these cease to control the cancer, the oncologist can either give up or continue radiation and chemotherapy hoping that any therapy may give hope to the patient. This is often false hope.[7,14] If given beyond the therapeutic dosage, radiation and chemotherapy may even shorten the life of the patient while decreasing his quality of life. However, radiation is often helpful for pain control.

All of Cameron's early 100 patients had had surgery and radiation as appropriate. Chemotherapy was generally not offered in Scotland at the time. The use of vitamin C without surgery or radiation was thus untested. Most of Hoffer's early patients had prior surgery, radiation and/or chemotherapy as prescribed by their oncologists. Some patients continued these therapies. Of Hoffer's initial test group of patients, Table 1.6 describes the results of the 36 patients who avoided radiation and chemotherapy, although 24 had surgery.

Table 1.6. Median Life of Patients Who Refused Radiation and Chemotherapy, Months		
Therapy	With Vitamins	Without Vitamins
No surgery	16	1.6
With surgery	68	8

These results are from a very small group and may not be typical. Vitamins appear to be better than nothing but this is only implied.

The government's recommended amount of vitamins is based on the requirements of healthy people. Sick patients need extra vitamins. Hoffer's success is at least partly due to a good diet and extra vitamins. Some patients have quietly added vitamins to regular therapies without the knowledge of their oncologist, but keeping everyone fully informed and involved is best. The author recommends full compliance with proper medical supervision.

Discussion

Regular cancer therapies are only moderately successful. Cameron's vitamin C therapy and Hoffer's multivitamin cancer therapies are reasonably well tested. Vitamin C is very safe, and its side effects are apparently temporary. A therapy based on work at the National Cancer Institute may explain why vitamin C, an antioxidant, can act as an oxidant within cancer cells. This mechanism applies to all types of cancer that take in excess glucose. This may explain why Hoffer obtained good results with 30 types of cancer.

The therapies of Cameron and Hoffer have not been given randomized tests and probably won't—for lack of money. Most oncologists do not study vitamins as cancer therapy and are not trained or allowed to prescribe vitamins as cancer therapy. Doctors knowledgeable about vitamins but not certified as oncologists can prescribe vitamins to strengthen cancer patients but not as cancer therapy. Thus two types of doctors may be needed for a patient's care and safety. Vitamin therapies may be given to terminal cancer patients under proper medical supervision.

Conclusion

Although Cameron's and Hoffer's vitamin therapies are demonstrated effective, many consider them to be experimental. Radiation and chemotherapies were accepted by comparison with historic results. Vitamin therapies, being very safe, can also be accepted by comparison with historic results. Patients choosing vitamin therapy should work with both an oncologist and a doctor knowledgeable about vitamins for their own safety and for best results.

References for Vitamins, Cancer and Hope

1. Hoffer A. *Vitamin C and Cancer, Discovery, Recovery, Controversy*. 2000, Kingston, Ontario: Quarry Press.
2. Stone I. Scurvy and the cancer problem. *American Laboratory*. September 1976:21-30.
3. Cancer Facts and Figures 2005. *American Cancer Society*. Atlanta, GA: American Cancer Society.
4. Hoffer A and Pauling L. Hardin Jones biostatistical analysis of mortality data for cohorts of cancer patients with a large fraction surviving at the termination of the study and a comparison of survival times of cancer patients receiving large regular doses of vitamin C and other nutrients with similar patients not receiving those doses. *J of Orthomolecular Medicine*. 1990;5:143-154.
5. Hoffer A and Pauling L. Hardin Jones biostatistical analysis of mortality data for a second set of cohorts of cancer patients with a large fraction surviving at the

termination of the study and a comparison of survival times of cancer patients not receiving these doses. *J of Orthomolecular Medicine.* 1993;8:1547-167.

6. Hoffer A with Pauling L. *Healing Cancer.* 2004; Ontario, Canada: CCNM Press.

7. Letter, A. Hoffer to R. Houston, January 18, 2005.

8. Cameron E and Pauling L. *Cancer and Vitamin C.* 1993; Philadelphia, PA: Camino Books.

9. Stone I. *The Healing Factor – Vitamin C against Disease.* 1972, New York, NY:Grosset and Dunlap.

10. Cathcart RF. Vitamin C, titrating to bowel tolerance, anascorbia, and acute induced scurvy. *Medical Hypotheses.* 1981;7:1359-1376.

11. Morishige F & Murata A. Prolongation of survival in terminal human cancer by administration of supplemental ascorbate. *Journal of International Academy of Preventative Medicine.* 1979;5:47-52.

12. Riordan NH, Riordan HD, Meng X, Li Y and Jackson JA. Intravenous ascorbate as a tumor cytotoxic chemotherapeutic agent. *Medical Hypotheses.* 1995;44:207-213.

13. Creagan ET, Moertel CG, O'Fallon JR et al. Failure of high-dose vitamin C (ascorbic acid) therapy to benefit patients with advanced cancer. *New England J of Medicine.* 1979;301:687-690.

14. Moertel CG, Fleming TR, Creagan ET, Rubin J, O'Connell MJ and Ames MM. High-dose vitamin C versus placebo in the treatment of patients with advanced cancer who have had no prior chemotherapy. *New England J of Medicine.* 1985;312:137-41.

15. Lesperance ML, Olivotto IA, Forde N et al. Mega-dose vitamins and minerals in the treatment of non-metastatic breast cancer: an historical cohort study. *Breast Cancer Research and Treatment.* 2002;76:137-143.

16. Stone I. letter to Albert Szent-Gyorgi dated August 30, 1982, downloaded 4/17/04 from http://nutri.com/stone/.

17. Benade L, Howard T and Burke D. Synergistic killings of Ehrlich ascites carcinoma cells by ascorbate and 3 amino-1, 2, 4-triazole. *Oncology.* 1969;23:33-43.

18. Agus DB, Vera JC and Golde DW. Stromal cell oxidation: a mechanism by which tumors obtain vitamin C. *Cancer Research.* 1999;59:4555-4558.

19. Chen Q et al. Pharmacologic ascorbic acid concentrations selectively kill cancer cells: Action as a pro-drug to deliver hydrogen peroxide to tissues. *Proceedings of the National Academy of Sciences.* 2005;102(38):13604-13609.

20. Boik J. *Natural Compounds in Cancer Therapy.* 2001; Princeton, MN: Oregon Medical Press.

21. Hoffer A. *Clinical procedures in treating terminally ill cancer patients with vitamin C.* downloaded July 1, 2005, http://orthomed.org/links/papers/hofcanc.htm.

22. Cathcart RF. Preparation of Sodium Ascorbate for IV and IM Use (For M. D.'s only). Downloaded July 1, 2005; http://www.doctoryourself.com/vitciv.html.

23. Hickey S & Roberts H. *Ascorbate, The Science of Vitamin C.* 2004; United Kingdom: Lightning Source UK.

24. Lamson DW and Brignall MS. Antioxidants and cancer therapy II: quick reference guide. *Alternative Medical Review.* 2000;5(2):152-163.

25. Stoute JA. The use of vitamin C with chemotherapy in cancer treatment: an annotated bibliography. *J of Orthomolecular Medicine.* 2004;19(4):198-245.

26. Quillin P. Beating cancer with nutrition. 2001, Tulsa, OK: Times Press.

Cancer, Nutrition and Survival
Late addition to book

Dr. Hickey* reports that glucose is the key to cancer growth and cancer control. The hundreds of types of cancer have one thing in common: they live mostly on glucose. Limiting glucose can slow cancer growth. Fortunately, glucose makes cancer vulnerable. The conduits that bring glucose into each cancer cell can also bring in vitamin C. Inside the cancer cells the vitamin C reacts and forms hydrogen peroxide. This oxidizes and kills the cells. Normal cells are not harmed by large doses of vitamin C. Regular cancer therapies should be continued as these are mostly helped by vitamin C.

Very large doses of vitamin C are often used to control cancer. Doses of sodium ascorbate as large as 100,000 mg/day are given by I.V. Researchers have found that adding other vitamins and supplements reduces the amount of vitamin C needed and this may allow oral doses of vitamin C to control cancer. Dr. Hoffer needed only 12,000 mg/day of oral vitamin C in his trial with oral vitamins A, B and E plus selenium and zinc. He obtained excellent success. Supplements such as vitamin E succinate, alpha lipoic acid, coenzyme Q10 and vitamin K-3 might decrease the needed amount of vitamin C even further.

* Hickey S & Roberts H. Cancer, Nutrition and Survival. 2005; Lulu Publishing.

The vitamin intake should be built up slowly and under medical supervision.

Diet is highly important because glucose makes cancer grow faster. A bad diet can ruin a good cancer therapy. Depending on the aggressiveness of the cancer, the ideal diet for cancer patients might be high in vegetables and those fruits that are not too sweet. Carbohydrates and sugar should be severely limited while red meat and saturated fats can be minimized.

Cancer patients can play a big part in controlling their cancers. Oncologists rarely prescribe vitamins at therapeutic doses. Other doctors can prescribe vitamins to strengthen the patients but all should work together for patients' safety and best results.

Section Two

Other Cancer Therapies

Coenzyme Q10

Coenzyme Q10 is a therapy that may be added to the vitamin therapy. Coenzyme Q10 or Co Q10 is a vitamin or vitamin-like enzyme that is present in foods and is also made by the body. Absorption varies from person to person. Oil-based gel caps allow better absorption than dry pills. Co Q10 strengthens the immune system and is basic to the energy production of every cell in the body. It strengthens white blood cells rather than just producing more of them. It helps some white cells to recognize cancer cells. Co Q10 reportedly can minimize high blood pressure, heart attack, angina, periodontal disease, lack of energy and obesity. Co Q10 also has cancer-killing abilities.

As you might expect from this wide list of helps, Co Q10 can extend the life of animals, probably including humans. In one experiment, one type of mice that rarely live longer than 104 weeks were used. Half of the cancer-free mice were given weekly injections of Co Q10 when they were 68 weeks old. That is already old for a mouse. At week 96, 70 % of the controls had died of old age but only 40 % of the treated mice. At week 104, all of the control mice were dead but 40 % of the treated mice were still alive. All of the treated mice were dead by week 150.

In one small test, 15 patients had hormone refractory prostate cancer and a rising PSA. They were given 600 mg/day of oil-based Co Q10. In 100 days, 10 of the patients (67 %) had shrinkage of the prostate gland size and stabilized PSA readings. Excellent. Therapies that work fairly well with advanced cancer often work wonderfully well for early cancer.

In Denmark, Lockwood[1-3] had 32 breast cancer patients whose cancer had spread to the lymph nodes. The regular treatment protocol included vitamin C 2850 mg, vitamin E 2500 IU, beta carotene 32.5 IU, selenium 387 mcg, linolenic acid (an omega 3 essential fatty acid) 3.5 gm. To the test patients, Lockwood added Co Q10 at 90 mg. Results were excellent in the 18-month trial, Table 2.1.

Folkers[4] found increased survival of 5 to 15 years in 8 case studies. Most studies of Co Q10 have been on the cardiovascular system and periodontal disease. Cancer is third in studies. Co Q10 appears to be excellent at strengthening the immune system.

Table 2.1. Lockwood's Trial with Coenzyme Q10

1. None died although 4 deaths were expected in 18 months.
2. There was no sign of further distant spread of the cancer.
3. Patients' quality of life improved. None lost weight, and there was reduced use of painkillers.
4. Six patients of the 32 showed partial remission.
5. For two of these 6, the Co Q10 was increased from 90 to 300 and 390 mg/day. After 2 months, x-ray showed an absence of the tumor in one patient. The other patient had had a lumpectomy that did not remove the entire tumor. After 3 months at 390 mg there was no residual tumor.

References for CoQ10

1. Lockwood K. Apparent partial remission of breast cancer in 'high risk' patients supplemented with nutritional antioxidants, essential fatty acids and coenzyme Q10. *Molecular Aspects of Medicine*. 1994;15 Suppl:s231-40.
2. Lockwood K. Progress on therapy of breast cancer with vitamin Q10 and the regression of metastases. *Biochemical Biophysical Research Communications*. 1995;212(1): 172-177.

3. Lockwood K. Partial and complete regression of breast cancer in patients in relation to dosage of coenzyme Q10. *Biochemical and Biophysical Research Communications.* March 30, 1994;199(3):1504-1508.

4. Folkers K. Survival of cancer patients on therapy with coenzyme Q10. *Biochemical Biophysical Research Communications.* April 15, 1993;192(1):241-5.

Flaxseed Oil and Cottage Cheese

Flaxseed and flaxseed oil seem too ordinary to be a cancer therapy. Yet there is strong evidence to show that flaxseed helps. Combining flaxseed oil with cottage cheese has resulted in a spectacular set of testimonials. For someone dying of advanced cancer, the combination has low risk, negligible cost, but great hope and a reasonable possibility of cancer remission. It appears that actual tests on a specific group of patients have not been reported. But if patients have advanced cancer, what have they got to lose? More important, what have they got to gain? Life!

Testimonials indicate that many advanced cancer patients taking flaxseed oil and cottage cheese can experience good pain relief within 2 weeks. Measurable improvement in the cancer size and blood cell counts can be expected within about 3 months, if the therapy is successful for a particular patient. Side effects are apparently negligible.

The procedure for using flaxseed oil, FO, is simple. For a 150-pound person, 3 to 6 tablespoons, TBS, of fresh flaxseed oil are thoroughly mixed with one-half to 1 cup of low-fat cottage cheese, then flavored to taste such as with fruit or honey, and eaten in one or more servings during the day. The success rate is unknown, but some reports indicate 90 % with many types of cancer including breast and prostate cancer. In at least one case where the patient could not swallow, therapy was started by an enema of flaxseed oil and skim milk.

There are important warnings. The flaxseed oil must be cold-pressed and kept refrigerated to prevent oxidation of the omega 3 fatty acid. In local health food stores, "Barlean's" is one brand. Storage life of the oil is 1 year in the freezer and 4 months in the refrigerator. Do not substitute any pills or processed or heated flaxseed product for the oil. Three TBS. of flaxseed can be used instead of one of the TBS of flaxseed oil if the seed is ground (in a coffee grinder) immediately before mixing with the cottage cheese. Do not grind more than will be consumed in one day. After the cancer is in remission, the above dosage can be cut, but FO and cottage cheese must be continued or the cancer is likely to return.

Dr. Johanna Budwig, M. D.[1,2] in Germany apparently developed and publicized the flaxseed oil and cottage cheese therapy. Budwig developed the steps of using very fresh flaxseed oil and mixing it with low fat cottage cheese before consumption. For some patients, she recommended a low sugar and vegetarian diet as well as FO.

Budwig claimed that cottage cheese is a necessary ingredient for cancer therapy and that without cottage cheese, flaxseed oil is harmful to cancer patients. Charles E. Myers, Jr., M. D., [3] also advises against flaxseed oil for prostate cancer patients. He cites several studies showing that flaxseed oil increases the risk of getting prostate cancer. If flaxseed oil promotes prostate cancer, it is not likely to control cancer. When asked, Myers did not comment on cottage cheese with the flaxseed oil therapy.

Some patients have taken chemotherapy or radiation with FO. Frequently the white blood cell count will go up or not drop as rapidly as a doctor would expect. Some of these patients have continued FO therapy only and gone into remission. Some patients who continued FO plus chemotherapy or radiation have *died* as reported by Cliff Beckwith on the internet. A possible guess as to the cause is that the FO improved the blood cell counts more than it strengthened the body's ability to withstand chemotherapy or radiation. Considering only the blood cell count could lead the doctor to give an excessive dose.

As a possible alternate, a patient may consider continuing the FO, minimizing chemotherapy or radiation, being sure to check frequently to see if the cancer is going into or staying in remission. Obviously the patient and the oncologist must work together for safety. Remember, vitamin therapy strengthens the immune system while chemotherapy and radiation weaken it. In addition to cancer, flaxseed oil and cottage cheese are reported by some to be good also for arthritis, cardiovascular health, diabetes, energy and impotence.

The effectiveness of flaxseed oil and cottage cheese has not been proven nor does the author know of a good demonstration. Boik[4] lists good technical references on flaxseed and omega-3 fatty acids. Karmali[5] finds that omega-3 fatty acids and flaxseed oil are beneficial in the control of DU-145 human prostate cancer implanted in mice.

Flaxseed oil contains 55 % of an omega-3 fatty acid called linolenic acid. Linolenic acid tends to balance the omega 6, hydrogenated and saturated fatty acids that we consume. Boik lists the following ways in which omega-3 fatty acid can help control cancer.

Effects of Omega-3 Fatty Acid on Cancer

1. Inhibits the development of colon and pancreatic cancers.
2. Inhibits the growth of prostate, mammary, colon and pancreatic cancers.
3. Omega-3 increases the fluidity of tumor cell membranes and thus their sensitivity to chemotherapy drugs.
4. Omega-3 fatty acid is cytotoxic to human breast, prostate and lung cancer cells but not toward normal cells when tested in cultures.
5. Omega-3 increase the amount of prostaglandin PGE3, which is good, and decreases the amount of PGE2. PGE2 promotes the spread of cancer to the bone, decreases survival and inhibits the natural killer cell activity.
6. Decreases new blood vessel growth, angiogenesis.
7. Decreases cachexia, or body wasting, which finally kills many cancer patients.

The following anecdotes are quoted with permission from Cliff Beckwith, from www.beckwithfamily.com/Flax1.html.

"In 'How to Fight Cancer and Win'[6,] an account is given of a young woman, 35, who had cancer so advanced she could no longer eat. She was given enemas of flaxseed oil and skim milk. In a short time she was able to eat and in 3 months she was home taking care of the family."

In another case from a man using flaxseed oil and cottage cheese: "the doctor said his bladder had crystallized and lost its elasticity. He couldn't stay out of the bathroom 15 minutes... The doctor said it was a condition he'd just have to live with. After taking flaxseed oil and cottage cheese for a while, he went to the doctor for a physical. ...The doctor examined him and said, 'Mr. C., you've had cancer in your bladder and it's gone. The bladder is elastic again and everything is back to normal.'"

"A friend of ours has an uncle, 72, who was badly off with prostate cancer and preparing to die...He got the information and began using the oil. We didn't hear for some time, but one day I saw his brother-in-law and he said, 'Oh, he's doing great! He's going to meetings and there's no more thought of dying. He's telling everyone about the value of flax oil.'"

Flaxseed Alone

Dr. Wendy Demark-Wahnefried,[7] a research professor at Duke University, had a prostate cancer patient whose biopsy showed high levels of pre-cancerous cells throughout his prostate gland. He was put on a low fat (20 %) diet plus 30 grams (3 tablespoons) of freshly ground flaxseed. Cottage cheese was not included. Three months later, his PSA had fallen from 5.9 to 2.7. Six months after the start, his PSA was 2.6 and a biopsy indicated a complete absence of pre-cancerous cells. Next, she worked with about two dozen patients who were scheduled to have radical prostatectomies. They were put on about the same diet. In 2 to 3 weeks, their average cholesterol dropped from 196 to 162 mg/dl. For those patients who started with a Gleason score of 6 or less, the average PSA dropped from 8.3 to 6.7. Pathological examination of the prostate after surgery showed beneficial changes, even in this short period.

The authors commented, "These data provide evidence that a flaxseed-supplemented, fat-restricted diet may have a biological effect on established prostate cancer which may be mediated through a hormonal mechanism... ." The lignan in flaxseed is estrogenic and may reduce testosterone as does Lupron.

Testimonials are generally a poor basis for choosing a therapy. However the cost and hazards are minimal with flax.

References for Flax

1. Erasmus, Udo. *Fats That Heal - Fats That Kill.* 1993; Vancouver, British Columbia:Alive Books.

2. Budwig, Johanna, M.D. *Flaxoil As a True Aid Against Arthritis, Heart Infraction, Cancer and Other Diseases.* 1994; Vancouver, BC: Apple Publishing Co.

3. Myers CE. *Prostate Forum*, August 2000.

4. Boik, John. *Cancer & Natural Medicine.* 1996; Princeton, MN: Oregon Medical Press.

5. Karmali, Rashid. The effects of dietary omega-3 fatty acids on the DU-145 transplantable human prostatic tumor. *Anticancer Research.* 1987;7:1173-1180.

6. Fisher W. *How to Fight Cancer and Win.* 1997; Baltimore, MD:Fischer Publishing Corp.

7. Demark-Wahnefried Wendy. *Cancer Communication Newsletter.* April, 2000; Duke Univ:7.

8. Simopoulos, Artemis and Robinson J. *The Omega Plan* (hard cover) or *The Omega Die*t (paperback). 1998; New York, NY:HarperCollins.

9. Gillian EC. et al. The effect on human tumor necrosis factor and interleukin-1 production on diets enriched in n-3 fatty acids. *Am Journal of Clinical Nutrition.* 1996;63.

10. Yan L et al. Dietary flaxseed supplementation and experimental metastasis of melanoma cells in mice. *Cancer Letters.* 1998;124(2):181-6.

11. Thompson LU et al. Flaxseed and its lignan and oil components reduce mammary tumor growth at a late stage of carcinogenesis. *Carcinogenesis.* 1996;17(6):1373-6.

Essiac Tea

Essiac tea as a cancer therapy is supported by thousands of favorable testimonials but no formal studies. Essiac (EE see ak) is Caisse spelled backward. Rene Caisse was a Canadian nurse who got the formula from an Indian woman. Caisse tested and improved it over the years. She was afraid that if she disclosed the formula, the government would outlaw it or make it very expensive. Eventually she sold the 4-herb formula to the Resperin Corp. She expected that they would develop and distribute the tea. They did not. Later she worked with Dr. Charles Brusch, MD, who was a physician to President John F. Kennedy. Brusch was able to buy the 8-herb formula that Caisse developed later.

Numerous companies sell Essiac tea, even though the exact or real formula is in doubt. Several brands seem to work. One published formula gives 16 oz of Sheep Sorrel Herb (Rumex Acetosella), 6.5 cups of Burdock Root (Arctium Lappa), 1 oz of Turkey Rhubarb Root (Rheum Palmatum) and 4 oz of Slippery Elm Bark (Ulmus Fulva) to make about 4 gallons of tea. Local health stores sell "Flor-Essence" brand in liquid or dry powder for about $25 a box. The box contains 3 packets which each make 32 ounces of tea. One box is enough for 2 to 6 weeks. For advanced cancer, some people start with 6 oz. per day and drop to 4 or 2 oz when the symptoms decrease significantly. Caisse recommended a maintenance dose of 1 oz. The tea can be taken in 2 oz portions somewhat before a meal or 1 to 2 hours after a meal.

Side effects of the tea reportedly are few and usually due to taking too much, such as 12 oz. per day. Possible side effects include aches in the lower back or head, flu-like feelings, allergy, itches or diarrhea. By all means, work with a cooperative doctor. Since a patient is likely to use other therapies along with Essiac tea, the doctor might want to check liver and cardiovascular functions. The doctor may be able to verify measurable results in 3 months if the therapy is working. Obviously a healthy life style is important. Stop smoking, eat your vegetables and do all those things your mother told you.

References for Essiac

1. Glum, Gary. *Calling of an Angel.* 1988; Los Angeles, CA:Silent Walker Publishing, ISBN 0-9620364-0-4.
2. Fraser, Sheila S. & Allen, Carroll. Could essiac halt cancer? *Homemakers' Magazine.* 1977;June/July/August.
3. Thomas R. *The Essiac Report.* 1993; Los Angeles, CA:The Alternative Treatment Information Network.

Melatonin

Ah, that wee sleeping pill that sometimes helps with jet lag. As a strong antioxidant, it is effective against two types of free radicals. It increases the expression of p53 in breast and other cancers.[1] Thus melatonin can significantly reduce cell proliferation. It modifies many cytokines such as TNF and some interlukines to help the body resist cancer.[2] Lissoni[3] found that 20 mg/day slowed cancer progression to 53% from 90% in controls receiving only supportive care. Melatonin was helpful with cisplatin-refractory non-small cell lung cancer,[4] brain cancer metastases and malignant melanoma. Lissoni[5] suggests that melatonin at 20 mg/day may change some prostate cancers from hormone refractory to hormone sensitive. Animal tests indicate that doses as high as 250 mg/kg are nontoxic.

References for Melatonin

1. Peller S. Clinical implications of p53: effect on prognosis, tumor progression and chemotherapy response. *Semin Cancer Biology.* 1998;8:379-387.

2. Neri B et al, Melatonin as a biological response modifier in cancer patients. *Anticancer Research.* 1998;18:1329-1332.

3. Lissoni P et al. Is there a role for melatonin in the treatment on neoplastic cachexia? *Euro J Cancer.* 1996; 32A:1340-1343.

4. Lissoni P et al. Randomized study with pineal hormone melatonin versus supportive care alone in advanced non-small cell lung cancer resistant to first-line chemotherapy containing cisplatin. *Oncology.* 1992;49:336-339.

5. Lissoni P et al. Reversal of Clinical Resistance to LHRH Analogue to Metastatic Prostate Cancer, Euro Urology, 1997; 31(2); 178–81.

6. Lissoni P et al. Endocrine and immune effects of melatonin therapy in metastatic cancer patients. *Euro J Cancer Clin Oncology.* 1989;25:789-795.

7. Lissoni P et al. A randomized study with subcutaneous low-dose interlukin 2 alone vs. interlukin 2 plus the pineal neurohormone melatonin...for advanced lung cancer. *Tumori.* 1994;80:464-467.

8. Mediavilla MD et al. Melatonin increases p53 and p21 WAF1 expression in MCF-7 human breast cancer cells in vitro. *Life Science.* 1999;65:415-420.

Aredia for Pain Control in Bone Cancer

Aredia (pamadronate) was initially used as a therapy for osteoporosis since it helped to prevent the loss of bone and frequently to restore bone mass. However, cancer loves bone and Aredia was found to relieve bone pain, prevent loss of bone due to cancer, reduce excess calcium in the blood, improve the quality of life for cancer patients and (at high doses) possibly lengthen life.

As cancer eats bone, two things happen. Pain is obvious. The other is that, as the cancer eats bone, the byproducts cause the cancer to grow much faster. Aredia, a bisphosphonate, is strongly attracted to bone. Aredia appears to coat the bone to slow down the cancer growth. Aredia is usually administered as a 4-hour IV.

The *Physicians Desk Reference* recommends doses such as 60 or 90 mg once per month for osteoporosis. Some cancer doctors give a small dose initially to test for adverse reaction, then 150 mg/day for 3 days and then 90 to 150 mg monthly. Since Aredia is more effective at slowing cancer growth than in killing cancer, it is frequently used with chemotherapy drugs. Most of Aredia is adsorbed on the bones where some of it remains for about 300 hours. The rest of the Aredia in the body has a half-life of about 26 hours. From this it follows that single large doses may be better than frequent, small doses. In large doses, Aredia may be effective against non-bone solid tumors and may lengthen life.

Aredia is apparently not effective against rapidly growing cancer. Most tests have been done with multiple myeloma (spinal), breast and prostate cancer. In 20 or 30% of patients, Aredia causes flu-like symptoms for 2 or 3 days. In one quite-sick man, symptoms lasted about 2 weeks. Lack of calcium intake caused pain for one person. Irritation at the injection point, nausea and a 1-deg.

C fever have also been reported. Aredia was successful at decreasing pain in half of the patients. It is also good at stabilizing or regressing cancer and at preventing bone fractures and spinal compression.

For those men who have prostate cancer and take Lupron or Zoladex, these hormones can cause osteoporosis. If they experience joint pain from the hormones, Aredia and Fosamax might help. This has not been tested. There are many bisphosphonates, with Aredia and Fosamax and Risedronate (Zometa) being the ones approved in the U. S. Zometa can be given in a 15 minute IV. Before starting Zometa, check to see if any dental work needs to be done,

References and Summaries for Aredia

1. Berenson JR et al. *New England Journal of Medicine.* 1996;334(8):488-93, gave multiple myeloma patients 90 mg every 4 weeks for 9 months. Half of the 392 patients also received chemotherapy. Aredia was helpful towards reducing skeletal events (24 vs 41%). Aredia also reduced bone pain and improved quality of life.
2. Clarke NW et al. *British Journal of Cancer.* 1991;63:420-423. Twenty five patients received 30 mg of Aredia weekly for 4 weeks and then every other month. Eleven of 17 patients with initial pain were pain free at the end. Five of 17 patients who had been progressing either stabilized or regressed.

3. Conte PF et al. *Journal of Clinical Oncology.* 1996;14(9): 2552-9, treated 295 patients with chemotherapy only or chemotherapy plus Aredia at 45 mg every 3 weeks. Aredia was advantageous in increasing the time to cancer progression (249 vs 168 days) and pain relief (44 vs 30%).

4. Coleman, Robert. *Am Society of Clinical Oncology Symposium.* 1998;16019 outlined 17 trials using pamidronate (10) and clodronate (7). Overall, there was bone healing in 25% of patients and a 50% reduction in pain.

5. Gucap R et al. *Archives of Internal Medicine.* 1994;154(17):1935-44, found that a 4 hour IV was as effective as a 24 hr IV.

6. Hortobagyi GN et al. *New England Journal of Medicine.* 1996;335(24):1785-91, used 90 mg of Aredia or placebo every month for 12 months. With 380 patients, the first occurrence of bone complication was 13.1 months with Aredia vs. 7.0 months for placebo.

7. Lipton A et al. *Annals of Oncology.* 1994;Suppl 7: S31-5, treated 61 breast cancer and 58 prostate cancer patients with 60 mg every 4 weeks, 60 mg every 2 weeks or 90 mg every 4 weeks for 3 months. Thirty mg every 2 weeks was not effective for breast cancer patients although the higher doses caused healing of the bone in 25%. For prostate cancer patients, these 3 doses produced a reduction in bone pain but no healing of bone lesions. The prostate patients may have been sicker at the beginning.

8. Lipton, Alan. *New England Journal of Medicine.* Dec. 12, 1996; treated breast cancer patients with 150 mg/day for 3 days and then monthly infusions of 90 to 150 mg/month. This large dose was well tolerated.

9. Tyrrell CJ et al. *European Journal of Cancer.* Nov. 1995; 31A(12):1976-80, treated 69 breast cancer patients with 60 mg of Aredia every 2 weeks for a maximum of 13 weeks. No other cancer therapy was allowed. Pain, mobility and analgesic scores improved in 61, 50 and 30% of patients. At 8 weeks, the improvements were 33, 21 and 16% for 40% improvement.

Megadoses of Vitamin C for Various Ills

Megadoses of vitamin C have a long and successful history of therapy for many sickness, Stone[1,2]. The following describes actual tests with humans. Dosages are actual rather than optimum. Unfortunately, success/failure rates are given rarely. Ills other than cancer are listed to show the broad usefulness of vitamin C.

Some doctors recommend vitamin C at 3,000 to 6,000 mg/day for healthy people. They may increase this dosage up to 40,000 or even higher during periods of high stress or disease. However the government RDA is 75 and 90 mg/day. This dose is based on preventing obvious sickness but not on optimum health. Most animals produce vitamin C as needed in amounts depending on their stress or illness.

We could get a dose of 5,000 mg/day of vitamin C, for example, by drinking 6 *gallons* of orange juice. Obviously, supplements are necessary. Supplements should include vitamins A, B, C, D and E. Note that A, C and E especially work together. Lieberman.[3]

Thousands of tests were run on vitamin C at low doses with only modest results toward cancer. Vitamin C is cheap at $10.00 per month for 5,000 mg/day. Vitamin C can usually be used in conjunction with other therapies.

TEST RESULTS WITH VITAMIN C.
Dosages are in mg/day, spaced, and for a 160 lb adult, often by IV. Vitamin C by IV or injection must be given as sodium ascorbate.

Common Cold: 1,000 to 3,000 as preventative, up to 1,000 per hour as needed by mouth for therapy.
Poliomyelitis: children, 1000 to 2000 mg every 2 to 4 hours by push injection, 60 of 60 cases cured.
Hepatitis: Children: 5,000 to 10,000, more for adults.
Herpes and Shingles: 25,000 for a few days
Pneumonia, infant: 4,000, injected, much more for an adult
Whooping Cough (82 % helped): 2,000.
Cancer, many types, over 700 patients at 3 locations: 10,000 to 20,000 mg/day, 10% to remission, 20% didn't live longer, 70% helped some, gave dramatic relief of bone pain to 80% of the first patients.[4]

Cancer, bladder: 4,500.

Leukemia and cirrhosis of liver: 24,000 to 42,000, single case, able to return to work, lived 21 months.

Pancreatic Cancer, 6 cm diameter: 10,000 increasing to 35,000. All pain and symptoms relieved. Cat scan after 9 months: no residual pancreatic cancer, died after 20 years at age 79.

Brain Tumor, 2.5 cm dia, confirmed by brain scan: 10,000 mg/day. In 2 or 3 months, brain scan showed no tumor and almost all symptoms gone.

Breast Cancer spread to bones and abdomen, bed ridden: 24,000 mg/day, much pain relief and able to walk again. Died after 3 months.

Cancer in both lungs, a smoker, labeled "hopeless and incurable": 15,000 mg/day. After 2 years, she claims to be in perfect health. X-rays show regression in both lungs.

Arthritis: 10,000 to 25,000.

Aging: 3,000 to 5,000 suggested.

Asthma: 70,000 .

Glaucoma: 2,000 or more,

Barbiturate poisoning: 54,000, one test.

Tetanus: 140,000 for 3 days.

Snakebite: 3,000, divided doses of 1,000, injected every 3 hours.

Burns, severe: 3 % solution, topically, plus 35 gm every 8 hours for several days, then less. Gave immediate pain relief and faster healing.

Gangrene: 5,000 for a few weeks.

Schizophrenia: 36,000, 10 of 10 patients improved.

References for Megadose Vitamin C

1. Stone I. *The Healing Factor, 'Vitamin C', against Disease.* 1972; New York, NY:Putnam Publishing Group. The book is out of print but located in the Carson Library, Lees-McRae College, Banner Elk, NC 28804.

2. Stone I. Scurvy and the cancer problem. *American Laboratory.* September 1976: pages 21-30.

3. Lieberman S and Bruning N. *The Real Vitamin & Mineral Book.* 1997; Garden City Park, NY:Avery Publishing Group.

4. Cameron E and Pauling L. *Cancer and Vitamin C.* 1993; Philadelphia, PA: Camino Books.

Section Three

Prostate Cancer Therapies

Newly Diagnosed

So you just found out that you have prostate cancer.

You can expect to live a long time.

This cancer grows slowly.

You have time to learn before you decide on a therapy.

On the day you were diagnosed, you didn't hear everything your doctor said.

There are many good therapies. Some are gentle.

For most patients, there are several reasonable therapies.

You need knowledge to make decisions.

For every therapy, ask what is the success rate at 5 and 10 years.

For every therapy, ask what are ALL the side effects.

What are the percentages for each?

What side effects do you hate? Are the side effects worse than the extra expected life?

Is a cure better than long term remission?

Vitamins and supplements have helped many cancer patients.

YOU decide which therapy, not your doctors.

But work with and inform your doctors.

Be an active survivor, not a passive patient.

As you learn more, you will have more hope.

Join a support group. Prayer is helping the author.

Diagnosis and Staging.

Testing for prostate cancer is sometimes complicated. Prostate cancer probability increases as men age. A few men will get cancer at age 35, especially African Americans or those with blood relatives who have or had cancer. One little boy got prostate cancer at age two! The author suggests a DRE, digital rectal exam, and a PSA, prostate specific antigen test, beginning at age 35. Repeat the tests a year later to establish a base line. An annual rise of 0.75 or less is good. The author recommends earlier testing than most people, because there are now gentle therapies in addition to surgery or radiation. Gentle therapies such as vitamins or hormone have often been effective and have delayed or avoided harsh, invasive therapies.

If either the DRE or the PSA is unfavorable, there is a 70% chance that cancer is present. A biopsy (tissue sample) is then necessary to determine if cancer is present and how aggressive it is. During a biopsy the doctor uses a hollow needle machine to jump through the skin and grab a small sample of the prostate gland. Six, 8 or 12 samples are taken to sample various parts of the gland. If a sample is painful, ask for a painkiller before the next sample. There is a small, perhaps 10 or 20%, chance of missing a cancer.

A pathologist then examines each needle sample to determine if cancer is present and how aggressive it is. The Gleason number is a grade of 1 to 5 where 1 is benign and 5 is very aggressive. The Gleason score is the sum of the two Gleason numbers. The score should be reported as two individual numbers such as 3+3 or 4+5. The first of the two numbers is the more important. A score of 3+4 or less indicates moderately active cancer. A score of 4+3 or higher is aggressive. The Gleason score is an indication of how fast the cancer may be growing. The stage approximates how far the cancer has grown, Table 3.1. The combination tells the doctor and the patient how hard to fight. The patient should demand a copy of the pathology report and the doctor's reports. Ask the doctor to explain words as necessary. A wise patient takes his spouse or a friend and a tape recorder to the meeting (inform all present of the tape recorder) where these test results are discussed with the doctor. Another person's recollection or a recording of the conversation helps assure accurate processing of this important initial information.

Table 3.1. Prostate Cancer Staging

STAGE (simplified) MEANING

A or T1	Cancer found by biopsy
B or T2	DRE is positive
C or T3	Cancer is in or nearly in the prostate gland
D or N	Cancer has spread, metastasized.

Therapies

There are many therapies, not just surgery or radiation. Let me list them in the order that they might be used and then describe them.

1. Watchful waiting with early stage cancer. This might better be called active watching. Diet and vitamin regimen could be helpful here.

2. Hormones. The side effects are objectionable but usually temporary.

3. Surgery if under age 70 or 75. The side effects can be bad and permanent.

4. Radiation, including seeds or brachytherapy, also has bad side effects that can get worse over the years.

5. Cryotherapy or freezing can also have bad and permanent side effects.

6. Vitamins as a therapy are new to most doctors and patients. Vitamins have negligible side effects, can be used alone or with all of the above therapies and often give excellent results.

No therapy promises life everlasting. Surgery, radiation and cryotherapy can often give a "cure." The doctor's definition of cure is for the patient to die from something other than cancer and have no obvious cancer symptoms. The patient's usual definition is to have no cancer cells anywhere in the body. Since cancer cells develop frequently (daily?) in everybody, the doctor's definition is preferred. The body, the immune system, kills most cancers before they cause symptoms or become detectable.

As a strong recommendation, don't wait for symptoms to develop or get worse. Fight cancer immediately. We don't wait until the flames come out the windows before calling the fire department. Also, follow the cancer by watching the PSA and usually at least one other marker. PAP, prostatic acid phosphatase, and CEA, carcinoembryonic antigen, are often suitable. PSA is not foolproof. Prostate cancer cells with a Gleason of 9 or 10 may generate little or no PSA, even though the cancer is growing. Also consider quality of life. Is the therapy worse than the disease? What is the success rate for a given therapy?

Which Therapy to Choose?

The patient should choose his therapy but with the doctor's advice and guidance. This requires knowledge and study by the patient for the best long-term results. Aggressive therapies like surgery, radiation and cryotherapy can have bad and permanent side effects. They can preclude other therapies. There is no single, best therapy for a given patient. Knowledge has not advanced to that point and may never get there. Much depends on the patient's willingness to learn, to work toward controlling his cancer, to get the best possible doctor for his chosen therapy. The patient must think positively. If you don't like your garage mechanic, you get another. If you don't like your doctor, his suggested therapy or his ability, hopefully you can get a new doctor or HMO.

As a concer patient, the author knows more about vitamins as therapy than about the aggressive therapies. He emphasizes vitamins and hormones. He is using intermittent hormone therapy plus vitamins with excellent success. He is in remission. Excellent information on therapies other than vitamins is available in Dr. Stephen Strum's[1] *A Primer on Prostate Cancer.*

Description of Therapies

A patient diagnosed with cancer, especially prostate cancer, has many options. The body has been fighting cancers for thousands of years and the body usually wins. Most people don't get cancer.

Most patients accept the obligation to help strengthen their bodies to live the longest and most comfortable life. Now that we have the PSA test in wide use, the patient can better select the best therapy for himself. Improving knowledge over time should also improve the results of the tests reported below. Five-year results are based on therapies and knowledge available at least five years ago.

Watchful waiting and Surgery

Active watching should be a time to learn more, to get second opinions from urologists regarding surgery, from radiation oncologists regarding radiation and perhaps from a medical oncologist with a broad point of view of many therapies. Aggressive treatments, even hormone therapies, weaken the body and should be balanced by strengthening the body. A good lifestyle is obvious but important: no alcohol and a diet low in sugar but high in fruits and vegetables. Fortunately, prostate cancer is one of the better cancers to have since the doctor can follow the progress or control of the disease by the DRE and PSA tests. These should be repeated about every 6 months. If a stronger therapy is required, it can be chosen and started.

Homberg[2] compared watchful waiting to surgery. Men with cancer contained within the prostate gland and a mean PSA of 13 or less were randomized in to two groups. Sixty percent of both groups had a Gleason of 6 or less. The 10-year test allowed a median follow up of 6.2 years, Table 3.2. Many doctors would not recommend watchful waiting to a patient with a PSA over 10 or a Gleason over 6.

Table 3.2. Comparison of Watchful Waiting and Surgery

ITEM	WATCHFUL WAITING	SURGERY
No. of patients	348	347
Deaths from prostate cancer	31	16
Total deaths	62	53
Erectile dysfunction	45%	80%
Urinary leakage	13%	29%
Urinary obstruction	28%	17%

In this short test, surgery appears to lengthen life and a longer test would favor surgery even more. Nerve-sparing surgery (to prevent erectile dysfunction) was not generally available during the test and is still not possible with every doctor, every patient and every HMO. Quality of life, a personal choice, was better with watchful waiting. If watchful waiting patients progressed in Homberg's tests, surgery was recommended. If surgery patients from either group progressed, hormones were recommended. All of these patients were retained in the study.

Surgery or radical prostatectomy, RP, is the surgical removal of the prostate gland and the cancer it contains. It is rarely done on men over 70. Most doctors do not operate if the cancer has spread beyond the prostate gland. Some results are given in Table 3.2. The ability and experience of the doctor are frequently more important than the choice between surgery and radiation.

The following comparison of various therapies, Table 3.3, is mostly from Dr. Strum's book. He classifies patients according to low, medium or high risk. He looks at 4 factors.

For low risk, the man would have at least one of the following factors: stage T1 or T2, PSA less than 10 and Gleason less than 7.

For medium risk, he would have two of the following factors: stage T3, PSA 10 or more and Gleason over 6.

For high risk, he would have all three of these factors: Stage T3 or higher, PSA 10 or more and Gleason over 6.

Table 3.3. Comparison of Prostate Cancer Therapies

Comparison of Radiation, Seeds and Chemotherapy

Percent of patients with low PSA after 5 years:

Therapy/Risk	Low	Medium	High
Radiation, 3D Conformal	85	65	35
Seeds	87	32	-
Cryotherapy	76	71	45

Expected Time of Remission with Surgery

Percent of patients with low PSA after 15 years:
Cancer in capsule 89%, Outside capsule 69%

Proton Beam Results

Percent of Patients with Low PSA at 4.5 years

Initial PSA:	Less than 4	4.1 to 10	10.1 to 20	Over 20
	100	89	72	53

Chemotherapy is not very good with prostate cancer because this type of cancer grows relatively slowly. Chemotherapy mostly works by killing rapidly dividing cells. If your doctor recommends chemotherapy, ask to speak to some of his long-term chemotherapy patients. After the standard treatments of surgery, seeds, radiation, cryotherapy and hormones have failed, a doctor might use one or more of the following chemotherapy drugs: Nizoral, Ketoconozole, Prednisone, Hydrocortisone, Estramustine and Etoposide. They add perhaps 10 months to a man's life. Chemotherapy greatly weakens the immune system. New chemotherapy drugs such as Tomaxofen for breast cancer may be helpful for prostate cancer. Newer techniques using dual chemotherapy agents may add 20 months of life. Progress reported in 2004 and 2005 promises much better results if these therapies become approved. Nausea, weakness, hair loss, pain and other side effects of chemotherapy may make the extra life undesirable.

The side effects of standard therapies for prostate cancer are summarized in Table 3.4.

Table 3.4.
Side effects of Prostate Cancer Therapy

Therapy	Surgery	External Radiation	Seeds	Cryo.
Rising PSA	22	80	9-19	80
% at years	3yr	5-9	-	5
Impotence:				
nerve sparing	30%	50%	-	-
regular	60-90%	50%	15%	80%
Incontinence:				
short term	60%	-	0-6%	-
@1 yr	3-43	-	1-4%	-
Other injury	5%	-	-	7%
Chronic diarrhea	5%			
Urinary obstruction	10-15%	-	-	5%
Chronic pain	-	-	1%	-

Table 3.5. PSA after Surgery—Variation of Results between Different Trials

Years	3	4	5	10	10
Percent with rising PSA	22%	28	85	30	59

The wide variation of results from these separate trials can be explained by the various stages of the cancer patients, the health of the patients, the definition of rising PSA and the skill of the doctors. Many will disagree with the numbers in this table.

For many or most of the above therapies, when the PSA starts to rise after treatment failure, one can expect several years before pain and then a few more years before death. Hormones are usually prescribed when the PSA rises and sometimes before.

Hormones

In 1996, hormone therapy was highly experimental if used as the initial therapy before surgery or radiation. Patients in 2005 were frequently getting hormone therapy as initial treatment. In 1996, almost all doctors though that hormones, once started, had to be continued forever. Now, intermittent therapy is popular and, hopefully, the most common situation. Table 3.6 describes the functions of the various hormones commonly used.

Intermittent Hormone Therapy

Intermittent hormone therapy, also called androgen deprivation therapy, ADT-2, is done by taking Lupron and (Casodex or Eulexin) for a period such as twelve months. This is the "on time." Then the Lupron and Casodex or Eulexin are stopped during the "off time." Proscar is added to ADT-2 to make ADT-3 and the Proscar is continued indefinitely after the Lupron and Casodex are stopped. Table 3.7 shows that 32% of patients taking Proscar had a low PSA even after 120 months.

If PSA rises to 5 (or 2.5 if on Proscar) then hormone therapy can be restarted, even several times. Hormones have significant side effects, however most of these are temporary and can be treated.

Table 3.6. Types and Functions of Various Hormones

1. Lupron, Zoladex and similar compounds stop the testes from producing testosterone. Prostate cancer uses testosterone to grow.
2. Casodex and Eulexin shield the prostate cancer from the testosterone that comes from the adrenal gland, a second step.
3. Proscar minimizes the conversion of testosterone to dihydrotestosterone, a compound that is 5 times as bad in making cancer grow, a third step.

The first 2 steps are called ADT-2 for androgen deprivation therapy. Adding Proscar makes ADT-3. *The different hormones in ADT-3 or ADT-3 do different things and can be much more effective if used simultaneously.* Another therapy is Casodex at 3 pills/day plus Proscar. Potency is usually maintained but few if any clinical results are available.

Table 3.7. Percent of Patients Still on Off Time

Based on patient "on time" of at least 12 months and with a PSA less than 0.1 during 9 months of "on time."

Months	20	40	44	120
ADT-3	70	48	32	32
ADT-2	39	21	16	0

Table 3.8. Possible Side Effects of ADT-2 or ADT-3[1]

Side Effects | Therapies

1. Osteoporosis,   Possible after 6 months on Lupron,
probable after 2 years on Lupron.
Fosamax, 1 pill/week
Aredia, 4 hr IV, weekly
Zometa, 15 min IV, monthly

2. Other problems

	Start @ months	Moderate side effects	Bad side effects
Impotence while On Lupron			95%
Mental/Emotional	1-2	+3%	14, stop Lupron
Bone/joint pain	2-6	26	4
Breast pain	>12	18	19
Use low-dose chest radiation if breast enlargement starts.			
Anemia	2-12	32	13
Hot Flashes	1-2	23	25
Use Megace or other Rx drug			
Weakness	1-4+	51	5
Exercise helps.			

After using Lupron for a year but not longer, testosterone and potency will usually recover in about 6 months and most side effects diminish or disappear except osteoporosis, breast enlargement and possibly hot flashes. With Lupron for over 2 years, testosterone may never recover. Using Lupron for 3 to 6 months will drop the PSA and shrink the cancer but will not kill much of the cancer.

Vitamins

For more complete information on vitamins, see Section One.

Selecting a Therapy

With so many therapies, how do we choose? Realize that each patient, each cancer and each doctor is different. And things change as we get sicker or heal. If we are relatively old, based on our health and lives of our blood relatives (not on our calendar years), just watching and checking may the best. Active watching means improving our general health and getting a PSA and DRE test every 6 months or so.

Vitamins to strengthen the body can be called part of active watching. Vitamins at therapeutic dosages can be the first step if active watching becomes inadvisable. Likewise, vitamins can be part of surgery or radiation or some types of chemotherapy.

Surgery is frequently warranted for younger men (under 60 or so). It is rarely used if the cancer has escaped outside of the prostate gland.

Radiation, external or seeds, is commonly used as the initial treatment or if cancer returns after surgery.

Hormone therapy, especially intermittent triple hormone therapy, is gaining wider use because side effects are mostly temporary.

Chemotherapy is common if surgery and radiation have failed. The quality of life is poor with this therapy and actual life extension is minimal.

Hormones plus chemotherapy has been successful for a few doctors: Leibowitz,[3] Bagley,[4] and Servadio,[5] as noted later.

Getting a second opinion from a doctor with a different specialty is recommended.

If Prostate Cancer Returns

Surgery, radiation, hormone therapies and vitamins usually control prostate cancer. If cancer returns (PSA rises) after these, there are several good options with more being developed. Increasing the vitamin C dosage almost to the point of diarrhea may improve the vitamin therapy. Other vitamins can also be increased. When regular hormone therapies fail with prostate cancer, the cancer is called hormone refractory. The first option is to stop the use of Lupron and Casodex or Eulexin. The cancer, which may have learned to use Lupron and Casodex as food, suddenly becomes starved. In about half of patients, the PSA will drop significantly for a period of 3 months to

6 years or longer. This is called antiandrogen withdrawal syndrome. Surprisingly, this is a cancer therapy that is easy and economical. Instead of stopping the Lupron, increasing the dosage may be helpful, especially if the testosterone in the blood is too high.

You can strengthen the immune system whether you have early or late stage cancer. You have stopped smoking, haven't you? Control your stress, get enough exercise if possible, eat 6 to 10 servings of fruits and vegetables a day and you are well started. A low fat diet is highly recommended along with a generous intake of vitamins and minerals. If you are too thin, some people don't recommend red meat because that puts an extra burden on the stomach.

Section Two describes therapies for cancers in general. These may also help people with prostate cancer. For example if pain occurs where the cancer eats the bone, local radiation is a good palliative. As cancer eats bone, the byproducts cause the cancer to grow even faster. Aredia[6] is very good at stopping pain, especially when used at a dosage of 90 mg infused over 60 minutes at weekly intervals.[7] Aredia[8] sticks tightly to the bone as a shield. It has a 26-hour half-life in the tissues, but some of it sticks to the bone surface even after 300 hours.

Several therapies are documented in small studies but not widely known. These therapies work by strengthening the immune system and several can often be used at the same time. Lockwood[9] used coenzyme Q10, CoQ10, at 90 mg/day plus 2,700 mg/day of vitamin C with 32 advanced breast cancer patients. In the 18-month test, none died although 4 were expected to die. Two of the 32 patients were then given 300 or 390 mg/day of CoQ10 and obtained complete remission. Fifteen advanced-stage prostate cancer patients were fed 600 mg/day of CoQ10 for 8 weeks,[10] a very short test. In 67%, the cancer shrank or became stable.

Green tea is extensively consumed in the orient where cancer is less frequently diagnosed. Tests on human prostate cancer[11,12] implanted in mice showed that green tea extract slowed the growth and decreased the size of cancer. Implanted cancers grew only about 20% in 14 days in mice given a green tea extract (EGCG). In the controls, the cancer grew to three times its original size. Therapy was reversed and EGCG was then given to the former controls. In 14 days more, their cancer decreased almost to its original size. For the mice started on EGCG, when the EGCG was stopped, the cancer grew to five times its original size in the next 14 days. Hopefully, green tea or its extract will work well in humans with prostate cancer.

The combination of chemotherapy and hormones has worked extremely well for two long-term tests. Bagley[4] used Velban, Adriamycin, Mitomycin and orchiectomy (surgery) with 27 patients and obtained outstanding results. After 5 years, there were 22 with an undetectable PSA level. Of the remaining 5 patients, three had a PSA less than 2.0 and two had PSA's of 13 and 33. Nausea and vomiting were minimal. No deaths were reported in the 5-year study. Strum[13] would modify this regimen using newer medicines and knowledge but he gives no results.

Servadio[5] gave cytoxan, 5FU, orchiectomy and DES to over 36 patients with advanced, stage D2 metastatic prostate cancer. Seventy five percent had pain relief, 50% had both subjective and objective improvement, 82 % had regression or stabilization of the primary tumor and 55 % had disappearance or stabilization of bone lesions as shown by bone scans. Most importantly, 58 % were alive after 5 years and 55 % alive after 15 years. This is wonderful. Dosages were fairly strong the first 2 years when compared to regular chemotherapy doses. On the third and fourth years, dosages were decreased and for the fifth year decreased further. Mild radiation was initially given to prevent breast enlargement. Strum thinks that the Servadio regimen may be over treatment, but the excellent results (considering the available knowledge 15 years ago) are more important.

Leibowitz[3] often prescribes Proscar, Taxotere, Emcyt, Decadron, Aredia and sometimes Carboplatin. Aredia is primarily for osteoporosis, but it is also known for pain relief from cancer in the bone and for preventing cancer from getting into the bone. In a group of about 16 men, 9 had a PSA drop of at least 89%, and 14 had a PSA drop of at least 50%. The author phoned Dr. Leibowitz's office, 310-229-3555, to get the names of 7 of his patients taking Taxotere and willing to talk. Three were called and the author was very favorably impressed with their successes. A South Carolina doctor was located who can use the therapy.

PC-SPES is no longer available. As a substitute, consider compounds called PC-Hope (on the internet), PEENUTS or PC PLUS at 1-800-860-9583.

Hope

My main message is hope. Compared to a few years ago, life expectancy and quality of life are vastly improved. Even without the wonder drugs promised "in a few years," we can live longer and happier than expected. Remember, there is much hope even with advanced cancer. Your doctor may not be accustomed to strengthening the immune system; so work with him, educate him if necessary. Find an additional doctor if necessary. Your life with cancer involves critical decisions, so be firm with your doctors about the medical choices you select. But you need him. He needs you.

Author's Regimen, 2/16/2006

Aim

As of 1997 at age 74, to keep his cancer in remission for 25 years.

Diagnosis

In March 1997 a biopsy showed prostate cancer with a Gleason of 3+3 in 1 of 6 needles, stage T1c. PSA was 8.1 but had doubled in the prior 6 months. Thus he had aggressive, early stage cancer, probably confined.

Therapy

External radiation was recommended but refused because of the side effects of possible incontinence, impotence and probable return of cancer in 5 or 10 years. Started Lupron and Eulexin. On 5/1/97 started Proscar at 5 mg/day to give triple androgen deprivation therapy, ADT-3. Lupron and Eulexin were continued for 13 months followed by Proscar only and vitamins during the "off" period. With study the author realized that he should greatly improve his immune system in addition to ADT-3. He increased his vitamins, did somewhat more exercise and decreased wine and red meat consumption.

Supplements

Pills are now about as follows: Proscar 2.5 mg, Vitamins: A (acetate) 10,000 IU, Beta Carotene 25,000, B complex 100; vitamin B12, 2000 mcg; vitamin C 10,000 mg as ascorbic acid, vitamin D 400 IU, vitamin E succinate 400 IU and a strong multivitamin which includes some of the these supplements. Selenium 225 mcg, calcium 1000 mg, Coenzyme Q10, 100 mg, mostly fish and chicken for protein, calcium 1000 mg, magnesium 250 mg, 2 or 3 bags of green tea, 3 TBS freshly ground flax seed.

Results

PSA dropped to 0.1 at 3 months and then to less than 0.1 until start of "off period" on 5/98. PSA rose slowly to 1.1 on 9/99. As of 2/16/06, his PSA had drifted down to 0.3 and leveled off. This is wonderful and probably due to the vitamins and Proscar. Bone density was good in 4/98 and better in 11/04. Good energy level and no pains since diagnosis. Mild hot flashes continue, probably from the Proscar.

Prognosis

Based on the above good results and Dr. Strum's report, The author expects to stay on the off period (Proscar and vitamins) for several more years. If PSA trends up, he would increase his vitamin C almost to diarrhea and take the vitamin in divided doses every 2 hours. If that doesn't work then he can restart Lupron and Eulexin. Please check back in 15 years to see how he's doing. Other things he might try, if need be, include flaxseed oil and cottage cheese, Essiac tea, more CoQ10, green tea extract and a more vegetable diet.

References for Prostate Cancer Therapies

1. Strum SB & Pogliano D. *A Primer on Prostate Cancer*. 2002; Hollywood, Florida: The Life Extension Foundation.
2. Homberg L et al. A randomized trial comparing radical prostatectomy with watchful waiting in early stage prostate cancer. *New England Journal of Medicine*. 2002;347 (11):781-789.
3. Leibowitz R, Hormone refractory cancer, www.prostatepointers.org/prostate/Leibowitz/leib20.html
4. Bagley C et al. Adjuvant chemotherapy and hormonal therapy of high-risk prostate cancer. *Proc. Amer. Soc. Clinical Oncology*. 1995;14:230.
5. Servadio C et al. Combined hormone chemotherapy for metastatic prostate carcinoma. *Urology*. 1987;30:352-355.
6. Hortobagyi GN et al. Efficacy of pamidronate in reducing skeletal complications in patients with breast cancer and lytic bone metastases, Protocol 19 Aredia. *New England Journal of Medicine*. 1996;335(24):1785-91.
7. Tyrrell CJ et al. Intravenous pamidronate: infusion rate and safety. *Annals of Oncology*. 1994;Suppl 7:S27-29.
8. *Physicians Desk Reference*. 2002

9. Lockwood K et al. Progress on therapy of breast cancer with vitamin Q10 and the regression of metastases. *Biochemical Biophysical Research Communication.* 1995;212(1):172-7.

10. Lewis, James. Co enzyme Q10. *Prostate Cancer Exchange.* July/August 1998.

11. Liao U et al. Growth inhibition and regression of human prostate and breast tumors in athymic mice by tea epigallocatechin gallate. *Cancer Letters.* 1995;96:239-243.

12. Strum S, *Prostate Cancer Research Insights.* 1999; 2(3):15-16.

13. Strum S, *Prostate Cancer Research Insights.* 1998; 1(1):9, 11.

Section Four

Two Anticancer Mechanisms for Cancer in Humans— A Review

Townsend Letter for Doctors and Patients,
June 2003;239:104-106.

By Reagan Houston, M.S., P.E. ©
Reprinted by permission.

Abstract

Recent literature explains why vitamin C has been both successful and unsuccessful at extending the life of cancer patients. Vitamin C at 10,000 mg/day was effective in the form of sodium ascorbate but not as dry ascorbic acid. The ascorbate solution oxidizes to dehydroascorbate that readily and preferably enters cancer cells and kills them.

However Abram Hoffer achieved excellent results with ascorbic acid. Hoffer found dry ascorbic acid with other vitamins effective at 12,000 mg/day when used with regular therapies of surgery, radiation and chemotherapy. Hoffer primarily used vitamins A, B, C and E plus zinc and selenium. The combination effectively combats the seven traits of cancer. These traits include defective DNA, improper proteins produced by the DNA, improper signaling within and outside the cell, angiogenesis and ability to metastasize and to hide from the immune system.

Vitamins make oncologic therapies less painful, less debilitating and more effective. In the last 50 years, Hoffer has treated 1,000 patients with over 20 types of cancer. In an early test his patients with regular therapies lived a mean of 2 months, or 28 months if vitamins were added to regular therapies.

Hoffer's vitamins should be tested as a group. Vitamins are safe, cheap, and presently available and have only minimal and temporary side effects. Current cancer patients can consider using Hoffer's regimen under medical supervision.

Background

Are age-old natural compounds currently applicable as cancer therapy? John Boik's recent[1] and earlier[2] books on cancer therapy provide an excellent background. He described dozens of natural compounds and how they relate to many types of cancer. Cancers have several traits or characteristics that are similar regardless of the type of cancer. These traits are listed in Table 4.1 with some natural compounds that are or probably are therapeutic.

Table 4.1: Cancer Cell Characteristics and Therapeutic Compound

1. Gene expression, mutation and proliferation:
   Vitamins A, C, D, E and selenium
2. Cell growth and death, cell signaling and growth factors:
   Vitamins A, C, D, E, selenium and calcium
3. DNA division and redox signaling:
   Vitamins A, B6, B12, C, D, E and selenium
4. Cell to cell communication:
   Vitamins A, C, D, E and selenium
5. Blood vessel growth (angiogenesis):
   Vitamins A, C, D, E and selenium
6. Invasion and spread:
   Vitamins A, B12, C, D, E and selenium
7. Evasion from the immune system
   Vitamins A, E, selenium and zinc

Boik believed "My central thesis is that the most successful cancer therapies will be those that target all of these primary events involved in cancer cell survival." Hoffer has run such a test.

Vitamin C

Controversy hinders the use of vitamin C. Ascorbic acid and sodium ascorbate are two common forms of vitamin C. They react differently toward cancer. Cameron[3] treated 500 hospitalized, terminal cancer patients who had failed surgery and radiation. Most obtained major pain relief in 2 weeks or less. His vitamin patients lived considerably longer than the controls.

Cameron's therapy was vitamin C in the form of sodium ascorbate solution. He gave vitamin C at 10,000 mg/day. Most patients initially received the solution by IV for a week or two. Then the solution was given orally. Patients who could go home were given a one-month supply. He made the solution by dissolving ascorbic acid and sodium bicarbonate (baking soda) in water or juice, Table 4.2.

Table 4.2: Sodium Ascorbate Solution

Ascorbic acid	100 gm
Sodium bicarbonate	48 gm
Water or juice to	600 gm

Sorbitol syrup (200 ml of 70%) can be substituted for some of the water. Take 15 ml four times a day with meals to give 10,000 mg/day of ascorbate. When refrigerated, the shelf life is about four weeks. Continue taking the mixture indefinitely.

Cameron describes a hospitalized truck driver with a malignant form of lymphatic cancer. After 4 weeks of vitamin C at 10,000 mg/day, he was back driving his tractor-trailer. A few months later, the vitamin C was gradually reduced to zero and his cancer returned. In the hospital he received higher doses and in three months was "perfectly fit and well with no evidence of active disease." He continued to be healthy for the next five years. Vitamin C appears to put cancer into remission rather than cure it.

In confirming tests in Japan, Morishige[4] reported on 124 patients. Those who took over 5,000 mg/day (range 5,000-60,000) lived an average of 233 days versus 45 days for those with less vitamin C. As reported by Stone[5], vitamin C was studied for cancer therapy in 1936. He used up to 42,000 mg/day "in a case of myelogenous leukemia, giving complete remission." The major side effect of vitamin C is diarrhea if the dose is too large or increased too rapidly. Nausea, gas, upset stomach and skin itch can also be temporary problems.

Tsao[6] reported that sodium ascorbate solution readily oxidizes in air to form dehydroascorbate (DHA), and other compounds. The DHA molecule is similar to glucose. Cancer cells avidly take in glucose and, being defective, also take in excessive amounts of DHA.[7] DHA is an oxidizer and can kill cancer. Cameron's tests in humans tend to confirm the small-scale tests of Tsao and Agus. Normal cells can control the amount of vitamin C they take in.

Vitamin C is not always helpful. Creagan[8] at Mayo clinic ran a double blind test of vitamin C at 10,000 mg/day. He gave the vitamin as ascorbic acid and found the vitamin did not help extend life. Cameron and Pauling objected to Creagan's use of patients with prior chemotherapy. Pauling apparently did not object to the form of vitamin C. In a repeat test using patients without prior chemotherapy, Moertel[9] found that ascorbic acid did not delay the time to progression of colorectal cancer.

Vitamin C as oxidized sodium ascorbate at 10,000 mg/day was therapeutic to humans with cancer.

Multiple Vitamins

Boik advocated multiple compounds rather than single compounds as cancer therapy. Hoffer[10] ran such a test beginning in 1977. He gave selenium, zinc, and large amounts of vitamins A, B, C and E to his cancer patients. His primary vitamin was vitamin C at 12,000 mg/day or more. In an early test group of 134 patients, the 33 patients who refused vitamins lived a mean of 2.1 months. However, the 101 patients who chose vitamins lived a mean of 28 months. At the end of the 10-year test, 48 of the vitamin patients were still alive but only two of the non-vitamin patients. The vitamin patients also had less pain from their cancer and no significant side effects from the vitamins. Hoffer asked all of his patients to continue working with their regular oncologists regarding surgery, radiation and chemotherapy.

Table 4.3: Hoffer's Regimen		
Type Cancer:	Slow-Growing	Rapid
Vitamin A	10,000 IU	50,000 IU
Beta-carotene	10,000 IU	5,000 IU
Vitamin B-3	1,500 mg	3,000 mg
Vitamin complex	B-50	B-100
Vitamin C	12,000 mg	to bowel tolerance
Vitamin E	800 IU	1,600 IU
Selenium	200 mcg	600 mcg
Zinc	50 mg	220 mg

The vitamin E should preferably be the natural succinate type. Vitamin D at 200 IU to 400 IU can be included based on Boik's work, the government's recommended daily allowance (RDA) and the work of Lieberman.[11] Hoffer sometimes included calcium and magnesium.

Hoffer describes a woman who had a pancreatic tumor two inches long. After surgery to remove part of the cancer, Hoffer gave her vitamin C to the point where she almost had diarrhea. This is called the bowel tolerance level. She tried 40,000 mg of vitamin C, but settled on 35,000 mg daily. He added other vitamins and supplements. She followed the program for 5 years before decreasing the vitamins. Eighteen years later she was still well. For pancreatic cancer, Hoffer's therapy is especially noteworthy because there is no known effective conventional therapy for this form of cancer.

Discussion

Is there some theory to explain vitamins as therapy? John Boik[1] lists seven traits that distinguish cancer. Ideally, a cancer therapy should be effective against each of these seven traits. All of the compounds used by Hoffer are in Boik's two books. Hoffer's regimen is summarized[12] in Table 4.3. The regimen is balanced because it fights cancer formation and growth at all stages. The weakening caused by radiation and chemotherapy is balanced by the strengthening from the vitamins. The regimen combats many, perhaps all, types of cancer. Boik's small-scale lab tests and theory are balanced by many years of demonstrated success in humans. The regimen has a balance of minimal risk against good but not excellent test work. Tests of the type desired by Boik have already been done. Even suitable dosages have been determined. Hoffer did not give exact doses because people are different, cancers are different, and dosages can change over time. Apparently vitamins and minerals combat cancer by strengthening the immune system.

Hoffer recommended that cancer patients start vitamins as soon as diagnosed and that those without cancer take one-half to one-fourth of the amounts listed.

Did Hoffer use the best natural compounds? Boik suggests several compounds that may be better. Boik repeatedly objected to vitamin C in large amounts. The vitamin has increased the mutation rate to help the cancer survive longer in animal tests. However Cameron and Morishige demonstrated that 5,000 mg/day or more is therapeutic in humans. The overpowering advantage of Hoffer's regimen is 23 years of successful tests. Although difficult to do, other compounds or combinations should be tested against Hoffer's results.

Safety

Many doctors object to their patients taking 12,000 mg/day of vitamin C. Are there test results? Cameron[13] gave 30,000 mg/day of sodium ascorbate to some of his long-term patients. Sodium overload was a problem but not excess ascorbate. Cathcart[14] has given 200,000 mg/day of sodium ascorbate short term by IV.

Vitamins With Radiation And Chemotherapy

Doctors question the use of vitamins simultaneously with radiation and chemotherapy. However Lamson[15] reviewed the literature and found 36 clinical tests using regular therapies and antioxidants simultaneously. Results were less debilitating and/or more therapeutic in 31 cases, neutral or "possible helpful" in 5 and adverse in no case. High-dose vitamin C can become an oxidizer and kill cancer by a free radical mechanism. Radiation and chemotherapy kill cancer by the same mechanism but also kill normal cells.

Summary

The single nonrandomized clinical test by Hoffer is not scientific proof. For current cancer patients, the question is not proof but "Can I use it? Is it safe? Will it hurt regular treatments? Might it help?" Hoffer's regimen includes surgery, radiation and chemotherapy. Hospitals and HMO's might investigate the possible savings by vitamin augmentation. The vitamins are exceedingly safe compared to regular cancer therapies. The probability of a more comfortable and longer life is high. Side effects and costs with vitamins are low. Vitamin C in the form of oxidized sodium ascorbate is economical and useful but less effective than the Hoffer regimen.

Conclusion

Current cancer patients can consider using sodium ascorbate solution or the Hoffer regimen under medical supervision.

Reagan Houston is a research chemical engineer in Hendersonville, NC. His prostate cancer is in remission. He is facilitator of a support group. At diagnosis 6 years ago, his PSA was 8.1 and doubling every 6 months. (A PSA of 0 to 4.0 is normal.) Instead of surgery or radiation, he chose triple hormones (Lupron, Eulexin, and Proscar) and Hoffer-type vitamins for about a year. He then stopped the Lupron and Eulexin. In the next 17 months, his PSA drifted up from 0.1 to 1.1 as expected. However, in the last 39 months, his PSA has drifted down to 0.6 and leveled off. He has never had surgery, chemotherapy, or radiation. Houston believes the low PSA is probably due to the vitamins plus the Proscar. Parts of this article were published in The Prostate Cancer Exchange. 2002: 22: 5-12, and reprinted here with permission.

References

1. Boik J. *Natural Compounds in Cancer Therapy.* 2001;Princeton, MN: Oregon Medical Press.

2. Boik J. *Cancer and Natural Medicine*. 1996; Princeton, MN: Oregon Medical Press. 42-147.

3. Cameron E and Pauling L. *Cancer and Vitamin C*. 1993; Philadelphia, PA: Camino Books. 31, 209, 162.

4. Morishige F, Murata A and Yamaguchi H. Prolongation of survival time in terminal human cancer by administration of supplemental ascorbate. *Int J Vitamin Nutr Res* Suppl. 1982; 23: 103-113.

5. Stone I. Scurvy and the cancer problem. *American Laboratory*. September 1976: 21-30.

6. Tsao CS, Dunham WB and Leung PY. Antineoplastic activity of ascorbic acid in human mammary tumor. *In Vivo*. 1988; 2: 147-150.

7. Agus DB, Vera JC and Golde DW: Stromal cell oxidation: a mechanism by which tumors obtain vitamin C. *Cancer Research*. 1999; 59: 4555-4558.

8. Creagan ET, Moertel CG, O'Fallon JR et al. Failure of high-dose vitamin C (ascorbic acid) therapy to benefit patients with advanced cancer. *New England J of Medicine*. 1979; 301: 687-690.

9. Moertel CG, Fleming TR, Creagan ET et al. High-dose vitamin C versus placebo in the treatment of patients with advanced cancer who have had no prior chemotherapy. *New England J of Medicine*. 1985; 312: 137-141.

10. Hoffer A. *Vitamin C and Cancer*. Kingston: Quarry Health Books. 2000; pages 85, 71.

11. Lieberman S & Bruning N. *The Real Vitamin and Mineral Book*. 1997; Garden City Park: Avery Publishing Group.

12. Houston R. A new look at old cancer therapies. *Prostate Cancer Exchange*. 2002; 22: 5, 7-12.

13. Cameron E. A protocol for the use of vitamin C in the treatment of cancer. *Medical Hypotheses*. 1999; 36:190-194.

14. Cathcart RF. A unique function for ascorbate. *Medical Hypotheses*. 1991;35: 32-37.

15. Lamson DW and Brignall MS. Antioxidants in cancer therapy II: Quick reference guide. *Alternative Medical Review*. 2000; 5: 152-163.

Section Five

Appendix

Suggested Reading

1. Hoffer A. *Vitamin C and cancer, discovery, recovery, controversy.* 2000; Kingston, Ontario: Quarry Press.

2. Cameron E and Pauling L. *Cancer and vitamin C.* 1993; Philadelphia, PA: Camino Books.

3. Hickey S & Roberts H. *Ascorbate, The science of vitamin C.* 2004; United Kingdom: Lightning Source UK.

4. Strum SB & Pogliano D. *A primer on prostate cancer.* 2002; Hollywood, Florida: The Life Extension Foundation.

5. The author's web site: www.cancertherapies.org.

Dr. Hoffer's Raw Data

Every day we read about things that are tested for cancer. What does test information look like? Frequently the test will show, for a carefully selected group of patients, that pill A will change item B in the body in a way that may affect cancer. This is an example of indirect evidence. Such a test can often be run in a few months and then published. Published comments on such tests often do not describe the conditions or important limitations. No wonder current opinion changes frequently.

Dr. Hoffer's patients were the first 134 cancer patients who came to him. His procedure was to offer to all vitamins, diet and hope. Then he followed the group for 15 years and reported who lived how long. His data is complete, direct and understandable. His test included all patients who wished to be included. He did not need fancy statistics, only length of life after they first saw him. Because he included all types of cancer, his results are summarized in Table 5.1. The reader can judge for himself if his cancer is included and if vitamins were helpful for his type cancer, by examining the columns for vitamin C dosage and months followed.

Vitamins lengthened the mean lives of all patients except for one of three stomach cancer patients. Vitamins helped patients with 30 types of cancer.

Table 5.1 Hoffer's Raw Data

Patient No.	Type of Cancer	Treatment	Vitamin C gm/day	Months Followed	Alive Yes/No
13	ABDOMINAL	NONE	0	1.1	N
128	ABDOMINAL	S R	3-6	11	N
46	ABDOMINAL	S C	12	15	N
49	ABDOMINAL	S	15	101	Y
24	BLADDER	S R	12	64	N
114	BOWEL	S	0	4	N
101	BOWEL	R	12	16	N
69	BRAIN	S R C	6	6	N
72	BRAIN	S R C	12	28	N
100	BRONCUS	R	12	10	N
8	CARCINOID	S R	0	1.5	N
60	CERVIX	NONE	9	116	Y

Table 5.1 shows the type of cancer, the treatment (surgery, S; radiation, R; chemotherapy, C; or none), the months followed after seeing Hoffer and if alive at the end of the 15-year test.

Table 5.1 cont

Patient No.	Type of Cancer	Treatment	Vitamin C gm/day	Months Followed	Alive YesNo
67	CERVIX	S R C	12	3	N
120	CERVIX	R	12	3	N
12	COLON	S R	0	0.4	N
78	COLON	S	0	2	N
30	COLON	S	0	19	N
15	COLON	S	2	79	Y
45	COLON	S R	5	10	N
92	COLON	S R	12	17	N
122	COLON	S R	12	44	N
95	COLON	S	12	74	Y
87	COLON	S	12	127	Y
80	COLON	S	24	13	N
22	EWINGS SARCOM	R C	12	111	Y
31	FALLOPIAN TUBE	S	0	50	N
17	GLIOBLASTOMA	S	6	15	N
70	INTESTINE	S	2	71	Y
71	JAW	S R	12	6	N
79	BREAST	S	0	1.8	N
81	BREAST	S C	0	2.2	N
7	BREAST	S C	0	3.7	N
115	BREAST	S R C	0	4.2	N
59	BREAST	S R C	0	6	N
53	BREAST	S C	1.2	9	N
25	BREAST	S C	1.2	23	N
61	BREAST	S R	1.2	40	N
10	BREAST	S R	1.2	70	N
48	BREAST	S	1.2	70	Y
44	BREAST	S R	1.2	95	N
38	BREAST	S R C	1.2	96	Y
117	BREAST	S R C	4	51	N
55	BREAST	S	4	80	Y

Table 5.1 cont.

Patient No.	Type of Cancer	Treatment	Vitamin C gm/day	Months Followed	Alive Yes/No
124	BREAST	S C	6	45	Y
36	BREAST	S C	6	58	N
62	BREAST	S	8	89	Y
5	BREAST	R	10	78	Y
133	BREAST	S C	12	16	N
21	BREAST	S C	12	22	N
82	BREAST	R C	12	51	N
129	BREAST	S R	12	57	N
118	BREAST	R	12	62	Y
88	BREAST	S C	12	73	Y
63	BREAST	S	12	74	Y
93	BREAST	S R	12	74	Y
40	BREAST	S R	12	85	Y
35	BREAST	S C	12	120	Y
20	BREAST	S R	12	14	N
108	BREAST	S C	12	6	N
83	BREAST	S R C	18	43	N
96	KIDNEY	S C	12	17	N
126	KIDNEY	S R	12	60	Y
50	KIDNEY, LUNG	NONE	0	1.5	N
64	KIDNEY-LUNG	S	2	28	N
102	LIVER	NONE	0	1.6	N
103	LIVER	NONE	0	2	N
85	LIVER	NONE	7	16	N
26	LYMPHOMA	R C	0	1.8	N
66	LYMPHOMA	S C	3	105	Y
121	LYMPHOMA	C	12	50	Y
11	LYMPHOMA	R C	12	93	Y
74	LYMPHOMA	S C R	13	113	Y
99	LUNG	S R C	0	1	N
32	LUNG	C	0	2	N

Table 5.1 cont.

Patient No.	Type of Cancer	Treatment	Vitamin C gm/day	Months Followed	Alive Yes/No
47	LUNG	NONE	0	7	N
33	LUNG	S	2	7	N
97	LUNG	S	2	39	N
54	LUNG	R	4	6	N
42	LUNG	R	12	6	N
51	LUNG	C	12	6	N
39	LUNG	R C	12	17	N
106	LUNG	NONE	12	17	N
89	LUNG	R C	12	25	N
1	LUNG	R	12	103	Y
37	LUNG	R C	12	140	Y
2	LUNG	NONE	20	14	N
57	MELANOMA & BRAIN	S R	0	1.9	N
3	MESOTHELIOMA	R	18	5	N
16	MUL.MYELOMA	C	0	8	N
125	MUL.MYELOMA	R C	12	48	N
4	OVARY	R C	0	2.6	N
65	OVARY	S C	0	3.2	N
113	OVARY	S C	0	4	N
9	OVARY	S C	0	12	N
29	OVARY	S C	1.2	30	N
23	OVARY	S R	6	126	Y
130	OVARY	S C	12	8	N
116	OVARY	S	12	12	N
111	OVARY	S	12	16	N
109	PANCREAS	C	0	2.4	N
58	PANCREAS	S	2	72	Y
28	PANCREAS	S	10	2	N
119	PANCREAS	S	12	9	N
84	PANCREAS	S	14 - 40	173	Y
110	PROSTATE	S C	0	1	N

Table 5.1 cont.

Patient No.	Type of Cancer	Treatment	Vitamin C gm/day	Months Followed	Alive Yes/No
112	PROSTATE	S R C	0	85	Y
34	PROSTATE	S	2	6	N
107	PROSTATE	S C	12	6	N
123	PROSTATE	NONE	12	10	N
134	PROSTATE	R	12	30	N
105	PROSTATE	S R C	12	61	N
43	PROSTATE	R	12	72	Y
98	PROSTATE	R	12	72	N
73	PROSTATE	S R	12	77	Y
131	RHAB.SARCOMA	R C	0	1	N
6	SARCOMA	R	12	115	N
132	SPINAL CORD	S	12	67	Y
127	STOMACH	S	0	11	N
68	STOMACH	NONE	12	3	N
56	STOMACH		0	4	N
14	TESTES,LIVER	C	0	45	N
86	THROAT	R	12	140	Y
76	UTERUS	S C	0	4	N
75	UTERUS	S C	3	10	N
91	UTERUS	S R C	3	149	N
19	UTERUS	S R	6	117	Y
90	UTERUS	R C	12	10	N
41	UTERUS	NONE	12	99	Y
18	VOCAL CORD	S R	12	150	Y

Index

ovary 4, 96
oxidant 10-12, 16-17, 23, 27, 31, 42, 85, 89

P

pamadronate 43
pancreas 1, 4, 96
pancreatic 1, 36, 49, 83-84
Pauling, L. 4- 5, 19, 24- 25, 50, 82, 87, 91
PC-Hope 71
Peller, S. 42
periodontal disease 29-30
Physicians Desk Reference 44, 74
Pneumonia 48
Pogliano, D 74, 91
poliomyelitis 48
Proscar 63-64, 70, 72-73, 87
prostate 9, 30, 33-37, 38, 44-46, 51-53, 55- 64, 66-70, 72, 74-75, 86-88, 91
prostatectomy 59, 74
PSA 30, 38, 52, 55-57, 59-60, 62-64, 66-67, 70-73, 87

Q

Quillin, P 17, 27

R

radiation 1-3, 9, 15-16, 20-22, 24, 34-35, 52, 54-55, 57, 59-60, 63, 65-68, 70, 72, 77, 80, 83-87, 93
Resperin Corp 40
Rhab. sarcoma 97
Riordan, Hugh 6-7, 10, 16, 25
Risedronate 45

Roberts, H. 14, 27, 91
Robinson, J. 39

S

schizophrenia 49
Scurvy and the Cancer Problem 24, 50, 87
seeds 54, 60-62, 67
selenium 2, 12, 30, 73, 77, 79, 82-83
Servadio, C. 67, 70, 74
shingles 48
Simopoulos, Artemis 39
skin itch 8, 81
snakebite 49
sodium ascorbate 2, 3, 5-6, 8-9, 11, 13-14, 27, 77, 80-82, 85-86
Sorbitol syrup 80
spinal 44-45, 97
spinal compression 45
spinal cord 97
Stone, Irwin 6, 9-10, 16, 24-26, 47, 50, 81, 87
Stoute, J.A. 16, 27
Strum, S. 56, 59, 70, 73-75, 91
Szent-Gyorgi, Albert 9, 26

T

Taxotere 70, 71
testes 64, 97
testosterone 38, 64-66, 68
tetanus 49
The Omega Plan 39
Thomas, R. 41
Thompson, L.U. 40
throat 97
Tomaxofen 61
Townsend Letter 77

Tsao, C.S. 81, 88
Tyrrell, C.J. 47, 74

U

upset stomach 8, 81
urinary obstruction 58, 62
uterus 4, 97

V

Velban 70
Vera 26, 88
vitamin A 2, 14, 82-83, 86, 88
vitamin B 2, 73, 83
vitamin B complex 2
vitamin C 1-2, 5, 6, 7, 8-20,
    22-27, 30, 47-48, 50,
    67, 69, 73, 77, 80-83,
    85-88, 91-97
Vitamin C against Disease
    6, 25
Vitamin C and Cancer
    1, 24, 88, 91
vitamin D 3, 7, 20, 73, 82-83
vitamin D3 3
vitamin E 2, 6, 14, 30, 73, 83
vitamin E succinate 14, 73
vocal cord 97

W

weakness 65
whooping cough 48

Y

Yan, L. 39

Z

zinc 2
Zoladex 45, 64
Zometa 45, 65

Do Vitamins Really Work?

The author describes two of his friends.

Bill was diagnosed June 30, 2003, with non small cell lung cancer, stage IIIB. The doctor's prognosis was 11 months maximum life. Two months later, Bill started chemotherapy and Dr. Hoffer's regimen plus many other supplements.Bill worked up to 24,000 mg/day of oral vitamin C plus 100,000 mg/week of sodium ascorbate by I.V.

In August 2004, a cat scan showed no visible cancer and the doctor said: "Continue your vitamins and supplements." In May 2005 the cancer came back and Bill had headaches. He started radiation and then narcotic pain relief. On June 20, 2005, Bill died in peace with no pain. Instead of the expected 11 months, Bill lived 24 months.

Hank was diagnosed in 1992 at age 80 with prostate cancer. He was put on Lupron. In 2003 he had colon and bladder cancer surgery. In January 2005 he had cancer the size of a golf ball and had lost 30 pounds in 6 weeks. He looked very pallid and "thought he was on his way out." In February 2005, he started Hoffer's regimen including 15,000 mg/day of vitamin C. In the next 6 weeks he regained 30 pounds. In April his doctor said: "Your vitamins may be helping you," even though the cancer was larger. By October he was off Lupron and the doctor said: "I think I put you on Hospice too soon."

On March 14, 2006, he had no pain from his cancer and went out for dinner and a cocktail with three friends.

Mr. Houston has composed a book of valuable knowledge in easy-to-understand language for the lay person. I enjoy sharing his research with my patients, who strive to enhance their nutritional armamentarium and quality of life.

—*Connie G. Ross, M.D.*